The Creative Matrix

The Reshaping of Psychoanalysis From Sigmund Freud to Ernest Becker

Barry R. Arnold
General Editor

Vol. 10

PETER LANG
New York • Washington, D.C./Baltimore • Boston • Bern
Frankfurt am Main • Berlin • Brussels • Vienna • Oxford

Andrew Brink

The Creative Matrix

Anxiety and the Origin of Creativity

PETER LANG
New York • Washington, D.C./Baltimore • Boston • Bern
Frankfurt am Main • Berlin • Brussels • Vienna • Oxford

Library of Congress Cataloging-in-Publication Data

Brink, Andrew.
The creative matrix: anxiety and the origin of creativity / Andrew Brink.
p. cm. — (The reshaping of psychoanalysis; vol. 10)
Includes bibliographical references and index.
1. Personality and creative ability. 2. Creation (Literary, artistic, etc.)—
Psychological aspects. 3. Anxiety. 4. Attachment behavior.
5. Psychoanalysis. I. Title. II. Series.
BF698.9.C74B75 153.3'5—dc21 99-17536
ISBN 0-8204-4480-4
ISSN 1059-3551

Die Deutsche Bibliothek-CIP-Einheitsaufnahme

Brink, Andrew:
The creative matrix: anxiety and the origin of creativity / Andrew Brink.
–New York; Washington, D.C./Baltimore; Boston; Bern;
Frankfurt am Main; Berlin; Brussels; Vienna; Oxford: Lang.
(The reshaping of psychoanalysis; Vol. 10)
ISBN 0-8204-4480-4

Contents

Acknowledgments

For their criticial readings of the entire book I should like to thank Helen Brink, George M. Johnson, John Ferns and Lani Glanville. Joshua Kendall greatly improved the book's clarity and cogency. Patricia Crittenden elucidated its use of attachment schemes. Kris Wilson-Yang's preparation of the text and index included valuable comments. — AB

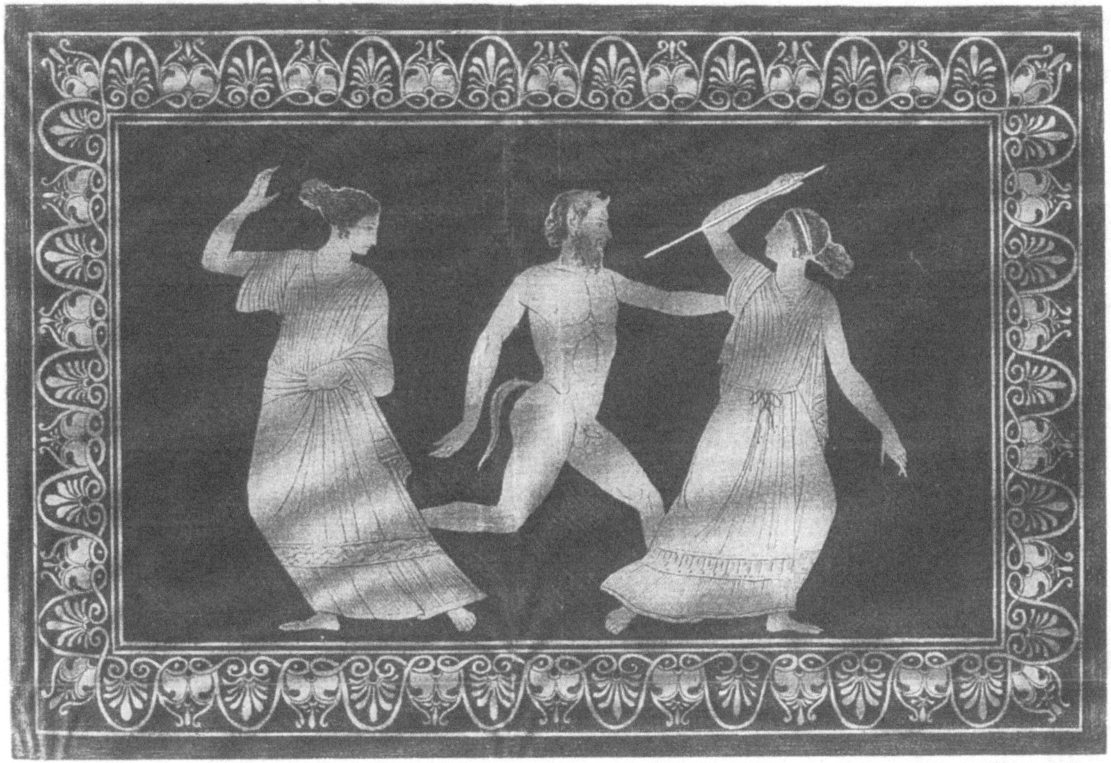

Allegorical Figures, *Collection of Etruscan , Greek and Roman Antiquities from the Cabinet of the Hon. W. Hamilton.* Naples 1766

Introduction

The Creative Matrix

Creativity as biologically programed adaptation to anxiety is generated in the developmental processes and reinforced by traumatic interpersonal relations. Creative adaptation to intolerable anxiety is possible for anyone, but it is most graphically evident in artists and writers who disclose personal and collective anxieties in their imaginative products, and propose "solutions" by discovering form amidst disorganized associations and feelings.

Basic anxiety is a product of attachment to imperfect caregivers at the start of life and, thereafter, to the persons in one's social network. Creativity consists of using symbolic means to locate and penetrate unconscious anxieties about attachments, to free them up and to reorganize them in formal configurations. Created objects containing anxiety tend to neutralize it and may improve accommodation to distressing experiences of attachment and loss.

Creativity begins with the instinctual attachment system which unites mother and infant at the start of life. Creativity differentiates adaptively, in response to anxiety, into the exceptional skills with materials, words and notes found among artists, writers and composers. Every artist or writer produces a personal iconography, primarily as a result of attachment-induced anxieties, only secondarily in response to social ills and injustices. Thus creativity links individual life with the symbolic orders of meaning in society and culture, but it starts with anxiety generated by a sub-optimal attachment style at the opening of life. To typify and understand anxiety-inducing attachment styles that necessitate, and answer to, creativity, is the task at hand. The attachment system is now widely studied in the life cycle, but little is being said about creativity as a concomitant.

To show the centrality of what John Bowlby and Mary Ainsworth called "anxious attachment" to creative endeavor in the arts, requires an excursion into early psychoanalytic thinking about human development and creativity. From Freud onward, creativity has been a leading topic of psychoanalytic theorists, as it discloses unconscious processes. Freud, and several of his followers and critics, made major statements about creativity using their assumptions about the ultimate developmental source of psychological suffering. As these assumptions have undergone dramatic revisions from Freud's time to our own, it is not surprising to find a corresponding array of theories of creativity. While there is no linear progression toward attachment theory as the governing developmental conception, something like it can be discerned when anxiety and its control are considered. We will thus consider the insights of Freud, Otto Rank, Melanie Klein, W.R.D. Fairbairn, Donald Winnicott, Marion Milner, Alice Miller and others, to arrive at a vantage point from which the importance of attachment theory can be seen. To this extent the book is historical and critical, offering assessments of theories of creativity before showing why a new one based on attachment theory is to be preferred.

Anxiety may be defined as unfocused apprehension of danger, a more or less intense chronic emotional arousal in anticipation of something bad happening. It usually anticipates recurrence of some traumatic insult to the attachment system. Anxiety is the background of fear, and it overloads the emotions threatening to paralyze them and to dislocate affirmative life processes. Unless dissipated, anxiety is trapped in the psycho-physiological system where it damages healthy relational impulses. Mood regulation associated with anxious attachments is thus a primary concern in achieving and maintaining a balanced, productive life.

The term anxiety in the sense used here emerged as the Middle Ages gave way to the Renaissance—the early modern era, with its increasing individualism and marked liability to depressiveness. As Rollo May wrote, Michelangelo's painted figures in the Sistine chapel have anxiously dilated eyes, as though fearing some judgmental nemesis.[1] Cosmic anxiety suffuses the seventeenth century French writings of Blaise Pascal, and it is strongly present in the English writings of John Donne and John Milton. Anxiety is the governing feature of the nineteenth century Danish Existentialist Soren Kierkegaard and reached its cultural apogee with W. H. Auden's *The Age of Anxiety* (1953), by which he characterized the twentieth century era of multiple revolutions and global wars. With the advent of psychoanalysis in late nineteenth century Vienna, the term anxiety acquired increasingly technical meanings. It may indeed be thought of as the leading concept in psychodynamic theorizing, and how lasting a developmental theory turns out to be depends on how convincingly it accounts for the genesis and persistence of anxiety. A theory of culture needs to account for the typical anxieties found in eras of history, and be able to trace their formation, means of expression and relief.

This study begins at the level of earliest human development, the individual sources of collective problems of social and cultural anxiety. It argues the need to understand child-rearing practices in any era whose cultural products are being studied. Of utmost interest is the incidence and kinds of sexual and emotional abuse found in the era under consideration. Whether typical anxieties in the arts are religious, social, or outright sexual, depends on styles of child-rearing that are open to historical investigation. The psychophysical effects of childhood traumas are probably much the same down the ages, but their severity and frequency change, as do the meanings given to consequent suffering. Overstimulation, emotional overloading and anxiety are perennial human risks, but their relative emphases change, necessitating careful historical and psychobiographical reconstructions. When does faulty attachment become "abuse", how is it encoded as chronic, unmitigated anxiety and what are the social and cultural provisions for relief?—these are some of the questions the study of creativity must try to answer. Research on trauma-caused pathological anxiety is just coming into its own—from the work of Bessel van der Kolk on Post Traumatic Stress Disorder to that of Richard Kluft, Frank Putnam and Colin Ross on Dissociative Identity Disorder—allowing more convincing reconstructions. But first the fundamentals of attachment, separation and anxiety (which invoke adaptive and sometimes reparative urges) need review.

Productive thinking about creativity was greatly assisted by Freud's insight of 1926 that anxiety arises in infancy with separations from the mother: it is a natural reaction to her possible loss. Anxiety is first a signal responsive to danger; it may well become "automatic" after repeated trauma or overstimulation, pervading the system with little likelihood of detecting, or reflecting upon, its origin. Since the organism cannot rid itself of anxiety, it devises defences against disturbing affects. As W. R. D. Fairbairn wrote, in simplified form these defences are hysterical, obsessional, phobic and paranoid and they combine variously, according to need. (Defensive strategies can now be more subtly classified, as will be shown.) Anxious attachment of infant/child to mother, or caregiver, is the background of each of them, but must be understood person by person. Containments of anxiety are never entirely successful, breaking through with greater clarity in dreams and chronic waking fantasies, and calling us back to their disturbing origins in faulty attachment. A range of disorders from shame and guilt-laden neurotic conflict, through more rigid character disorders, to disabling psychoses, is possible and, as flexibility diminishes, so does imaginative capacity to reflect on the origins of distress. But the urge to discover and integrate the origins of distress is never entirely lost, however seriously incapacitated. Thus the argument is that "creativity" is a biologically founded capacity ready to counteract anxiety at its source, though mainly outside conscious awareness. The mind has an inbuilt means of retrieving, re-balancing and integrating dissonant information that originates in early stress and trauma, and the consequent deflection of developmental pathways. Frequently distorted itself, thwarted and misdirected by life-events, the creative capacity is nonetheless a natural feature of the human organism. Its presence and promise have yet to be fully appreciated.

Creativity is traceable to the very start of life. A reliable maternal breast (or bottle feeding) is necessary for there to be aesthetic experience. Reliable nurture, especially in breast-feeding, produces healthy infants and, with the advent of attachment around six months, reliable mother-infant contact —including eye contact—prepares for life-long secure attachment. For there to be positive aesthetic experience later on, some experience of secure attachment is necessary, as well as some insecurity, for the creative urge to come into play. In other words, the sense of security must not have been too seriously disrupted for imaginative repair functions to operate. If early fusion or merger experiences with the breast are to lead to later aesthetic urges, they cannot be severely unpredictable or disorganized. If anxiety, alarm and confusion are too much a part of early experience, there is no ultimate security to re-access in the symbolisms of wonder and bliss.

The origin of the creative urge, together with aesthetic pleasure, is surely the "holding" of secure attachment, but a holding that knows the peril of loss and/or impingement. Maternal nurture cannot but be discontinuous and to some degree frustrating, with some level of anxiety in the infant inevitable. The question is: how did the anxiety arise that made aesthetic return to at-oneness so desirable yet problematic? Although severe bipolar disorder and creativity will be considered, our question is less with psychopathology as such as with the "normal" range of anxieties which need regulation. Mood regulation, the management of anxiety and incipient depression, is the main consideration, with attachment theory putting in perspective the overly dramatic attributions to artists and writers of "madness". Counteracting depressiveness is a central consideration in creativity, traced here to under- or over-stimulation, beginning at the breast. While mainly following recent work in attachment theory in accounting for creativity and the aesthetic response (for instance a study of smiling by Robert Emde[2] and by John Bowlby[3]), it is well to recognize that psychoanalysts have speculated usefully on the infant's experience of the breast as a precursor of aesthetic reactions. Some of this opinion is worth sampling. For the analyst Donald Meltzer, a newly arrived baby gives its mother an aesthetic "blow" of awe and wonder, as does her presence deliver a similar "blow" to the baby. Each impinges on the other, with a need for "tolerance" to control the inherent anxiety.[4] A more or less trusting emotional field develops, mainly from the mother's voice which "is the most evocative and carries the first aesthetic impact".[5] Later Meltzer wrote of "The thinking breast, the assimilation of the mother's eyes to her nipples, the function of her reverie in making available to the baby the food for thought . . .".[6] For Meltzer, arousal and control of anxiety are inherent in "The Apprehension of Beauty". Lenato J. Almansi in "The Face Breast Equation", develops the ideas of René Spitz that at about three months the infant deprived of the nipple redirects attention to the breast; upon frustration, an "I", "not-I" differentiation arises. With incipient "Iness", the baby sees the breast as "not I", looking at its mother's breasts which seem to look back, initiating identifications and projections.[7] Unlike Meltzer, Almansi does not attribute aesthetic experience to this primal differentiation, but he does help to account for original anxiety as a function of looking and seeing what cannot be had. So powerful is the original nursing experience that it remains encoded and, according to O. Isakower, just before sleep, adults may experience the breast almost hypnogogically as a soft mass imagined to move toward the face.[8] Writing of recent radical experiments with form, the art critic Peter Fuller remarked: "It was almost as if the painter had to go back to experiences at the breast . . . in order to find again, in a new way, his relationship to others and the world".[9]

Whatever may be true of re-experiencing the breast as an exciting and comforting aesthetic object, there is no doubt that the mother's face has such a function. Jerome D. Oremland writes, "The basic symmetry of the human face may provide the formal organizing principle to which all subsequent visual events are referenced. . . . In short, the formal matrix of all art may be the symmetry integral to the body image, and more basically, the mother's face".[10] The baby attends to the mother's changing facial expressions, knowing that her face always returns to symmetry. Daniel N. Stern points out that the visual-motor system in infants functions very early in development and that, in the three- to six-month period, interaction between mother and infant is carried out principally by gaze behavior. Experiments show that infants self-regulate stimulation by shifting gaze to and away from mother—a finding in keeping with attachment research.[11]

Allan N. Schore shows how the neurophysiology of infants develops through facial recognition of their mothers and the mothers' response to infants' signals. He writes, "the infant creates a schema of the face of the attachment object. This representational model contains a permanent abstract prototype of the mother's emotionally expressive facial expressions that is linked to the child's interceptive response to this input".[12] According to Mary Ainsworth and Mary Main, infants' representational attachment models of their mothers resolve into three general categories, within which are shades of variation: secure, anxious-ambivalent and avoidant, to which a fourth was later added, the disorganized. In the non-secure attachment styles, the governing concept is anxiety about lack of security. In anxious-ambivalent and avoidant attachment, but much less in disorganized, definite defensive, adaptive and sometimes genuinely reparative strategies can be discerned. It is these a new theory of creativity needs to consider in the light of improved understanding of regulation of infants' and children's arousal levels by "interactive repair" between mother and infant.[13]

Put at its simplest, if there is free reciprocity between infant and mother, with no (or infrequent) unendurable deficit or surfeit of stimulation, repair of separation anxiety by eye contact, verbalization and holding is uncomplicated. It is a natural function of mother-infant interaction, with mother taking the primary role as reparative agent. But in stressful attachments adaptive strategies are "created" by the infant to attempt to "repair" what cannot be corrected interactively. This throws emphasis on the infant's own self–protective resources, increasing isolation and self-holding in anxious readiness for the next assault upon its integrity. However put, an interior picture of the world builds up "imaginatively", or in a more technical psychodynamic language, assumptive models of reality, complete with alert defences against intolerable anxiety, are constructed because there is no escape from life as attachment. Ability to self-regulate arousal level is basic to the maintenance of life, and any saving strategy, even disorganization, a likely outcome of severe or repeated trauma, is better than complete loss of attachment portending death.

The research leading to this conclusion will be reviewed; here it is enough to say that work to date points to the most effective creativity occurring within a defensive framework combining avoidance with controlling defensive strategies (A/C). This has implications for understanding why bipolar disorder (manic–depression) has been found so often among creative writers. The question will be raised as to whether bipolar disorder may not be developmentally interactive in origin, rather than due to a primary biochemical lesion. Avoidant/controlling ambivalence can itself be defensively entrapping, and the creative urge, among those fortunate enough to have talent and energy, is an attempt to transcend its contraries. By transcend I mean that art displaces contrasting impulses into a language of imagery where they can be formally harmonized.

The following study does not find creative art to be a panacea for human psychological ills. It does, however, argue strongly for the creative impulse, leading to artistic productivity, being our most valuable and hopeful resource. Outcomes of high artistic creativity in improved relationships in life are exceedingly scarce, as every reader of the biographies of celebrated artists already knows. It is too late for romantic apologies for sensational but maladaptive behaviors by artists in history, but it is now possible to better understand them and to distinguish the creative impulse from misguided exploits. Emotionally "transformative" or "mutative" experiences are likely to be reserved for persons willing to pursue psychodynamic treatments, complete with transferences to an analyst; they are not so likely in the narcissistically engrossing pursuits of artistic creativity. But by the same token, it is important that the products of authentic art (that communicating unconscious wishes and defences) be understood in a new way: as simulating anxious attachments and their externalized formal resolutions.

To put it at its most general, pictures may be looked at for the moods of mother's face, recreated and transformed in displaced imagery—the artist's mother's moods, and our own, the viewer's, being reenacted. Any painting, not just portrayals of women, conveys conditions of mood in which anxiety has been recognized and contained. Similarly, the basic story of literary narratives is that of primary attachment, loss and consequent anxiety reworked in the light of accommodations, compensations and consolations. The archetypal story of man and woman's fall from grace into error, wandering, penitential reunion with their creator and redemption by faith and good works is essentially one of attachment, separation (loss) and regenerative 'repair' of the effects of the aloneness of that separation. I believe that if, beyond all their complicated elaboration, these basic biological encodings are acknowledged in the arts, we will be better served by the creative impulse, wherever it arises, to communicate and to receive from others their communications about innermost experiences of attachment. Imagination exists to discover and repair anxious attachments. At its most powerful it reaches back into the earliest formative experiences, amalgamating them with later relational anxieties in the creative matrix.

The theory advanced here is that creativity and the aesthetic experience of nature and created objects regulate moods, controlling anxiety and reducing the likelihood of depression. Central to the adaptive repertoire of humans, creativity should no longer be seen as the exclusive possession of certain gifted persons. This is not to question talent and genius, only to point out that the original creative impulse is simply human. Creativity belongs to the homeostatic system at the psychological end of the range of self-regulating functions built into the human organism.

It is not new to view creativity as adaptive; most recent writing on the subject sees it this way. Lacking is a biological foundation for theory which has become sophisticated but without the grounding supplied here. There is ample precedent for placing creativity in a framework of evolutionary and developmental biology, linking it to the control of anxiety. For instance, Parker E. Lichtenstein's "Genius as Productive Neurosis" proposes reduction of anxiety as a primary source of creativity.[14] From the "Panel on Creativity" of the 27th International Psychoanalytic Congress in 1971 to Gilbert J.

Rose's "Affect: A Biological Taproot of Art", a view of creativity as biologically founded has become established. Rose writes that "By providing a channel for symbolic repetition and re-experiencing, art continues the function of early mothering: its holding presence and containment of reliably balanced tension and release encourage affects to build up with modulated intensity and thus continue to differentiate".[15] In *Necessary Illusion: Art as Witness*, Rose shows further how creative art is a symbolic regulator of tension and release simulating the mother-infant relationship, but there is no mention of Bowlby's demonstration of instinctual attachment. For Rose, "Art may reactivate early motivational processes by providing an illusion of responsiveness linked to internal objects. Basically this means that art may promote emotional development by advancing the biological functions of early mothering together with the attunement and resonance inherent in this".[16] For attachment theorists, the psychoanalytic term 'internal objects' is needlessly vague. It is replaced by more precise descriptors of the consequences for infants of developmental interactions with their caregivers. As will be seen, new research, especially by Mary Main and Patricia Crittenden, refines the categories of adaptive strategies in which productive creativity may be expected.

Susan Kavaler-Adler's *The Compulsion to Create: A Psychoanalytic Study of Women Artists* takes a more skeptical view of creativity than do Rose's studies. Kavaler-Adler is a penetrating psychobiographer who measures the contribution of creativity to mental health according to evidence for its relief of suffering. Her post-Freudian object relations orientation produces new achievements in exacting psychobiography—from the Brontë sisters to Sylvia Plath. Her statement is "Old and widespread myths about reparation through the creative process and new myths in which artists' narcissistic fantasies are taken at face value and turned into theoretical fantasies force me to take a skeptical view of the prospects for self-integration through engagement solely with the creative process".[17] Kavaler-Adler's critical tough- mindedness is justified in an area where sentimentality and opinion have ruled too long. Object relations theory, stimulated by the writings of Ronald Fairbairn and later Donald Winnicott, gave new power to investigations of the child's inner world of imagination, as constituted from internalized persecutory maternal objects. Following their lead, Kavaler-Alder reveals intensities of inner persecution, 'false self' narcissism and grandiose compensation in her subjects not generally noticed by conventional biographers. As illustrated by several cases, when traumatic damage is pre-oedipal, the prognosis is poor for repair by artistic creativity. Kavaler-Adler concludes: "After reviewing the women authors of this book, it appears that the creative process cannot transcend developmental limitations".[18] The stark conclusion that "pathological mourning leads to an addiction to creativity itself, a syndrome I address as 'the compulsion to create'" must stand, but this may be placing too narrow a construction on creativity as a psychobiological phenomenon.[19] Although she has read Bowlby's work on attachment, she makes little of its broad application to the question of creativity. Bowlby's exacting attachment model of development is proposed in the hope that it will take us beyond the insights produced by object relations. That is to say, studies of mother–infant interaction by Bowlby and his associates introduce much greater precision into assessing the corrective capability of creativity. The problem for attachment theorists—who usually work with living subjects—is to supply sufficient developmental data to reach conclusions. Studies of persons who become artists are so far lacking. The intuitive element in psychobiography is valuable, and it can be strengthened beyond clinical experience by experimental findings in attachment research. I am thus delineating a promising field of enquiry following directly upon the insights of psychoanalysis, correcting and refining them.

Creativity is probably a late product of evolution, and certainly underdeveloped, but its presence is a hopeful sign of emergent adaptive powers, a sort of natural self-management of dissonant information. Creativity exists to counteract the disintegrating effects of traumatic threats to the attachment system and anxiety about such threats. In other words, the creative impulse to symbolize and externalize anxiety by re-processing dissonant information more consciously is allied to the "hidden regulators" being discovered (by Myron Hofer and others) in studying survival techniques of very young mammals. Creativity thus helps to relieve high anxiety about personal safety and survival arising when social support is under assault. It is allied to dreaming and arises from the same intrapsychic pressures to process dissonant information. Words, images and musical notes are the symbolic carriers of states of feeling needing reprocessing to confer reassuring meaning upon them. They are essential to the formal integration of confusing, sometimes life-threatening experiences and are the reparative elements of culture. To establish this claim for creativity the following propositions will be examined: (1) that creativity is an attachment phenomenon; (2) that the origin and nature of creativity is found in the anxieties of infant and child development; and (3) that studies of the creative arts need psycho-biological re-orientation.

To support the claims for the centrality of attachment theory, there follows in Part I, a review of concepts, and a history of their development through psychoanalysis. Part II comprises studies on the role of anxiety in creativity as understood by leading psychoanalysts. Its chapters form a brief history of how analysts from Freud and Rank onward have seen creativity. While John Bowlby's departure from the main tenets of psychoanalysis necessitates rethinking creativity, there is much in earlier views of creativity on which to build. To redirect debate about the adaptive function of creativity, in Part III a review is offered of the arguments especially of Nancy Andreasen and Kay Jamison, who study bipolar disorder in creative persons. Andreasen and Jamison are behaviorial scientists whose methodologies are designed to overcome the limitations of psychoanalysis; yet their "biological" orientation has severe drawbacks. A critique of their work from the point of view of attachment theory shows neglected "biological" considerations. The chapter entitled "Three Bipolar Poets" (Robert Lowell, Anne Sexton and Sylvia Plath) applies attachment theory in biographical examples to illustrate an expanded biological theory of creativity.

Notes

1. Rollo May, *The Meaning of Anxiety* (New York: Ronald Press, 1950), pp.162, 165; *Dictionary of National Biography*, vol. 1, pp. 538–39.

2. Robert N. Emde et al., *Emotional Expression in Infancy: A Biobehavorial Study*, *Psychological Issues*, 10, no.1, Monograph 37 (New York: International Universities Press,1974).

3. John Bowlby, *Attachment and Loss* (London: Hogarth Press,1969), vol. 1, *Attachment*, pp. 280f.

4. Donald Meltzer, *The Apprehension of Beauty* (Perthshire: The Clunie Press, 1988), p. 57.

5. Ibid., p. 60.

6. Ibid., p.135.

7. Lenato J. Almasi, "The Face-Breast Equation," *Journal of the American Psychoanalytic Association*, 8 (1960): 43–69.

8. O.Isakower, "A Contribution to Patho-psychology of Phenomena Associated With Falling Asleep," *International Journal of Psycho-Analysis*, 19, no.138 (1938): 331–45.

   In "Deep Calling unto Deep: Artistic Creativity and the Maternal Object" Kenneth Wright cogently offers a theory based on the "social" interaction of infant and mother. "I suggest that *in the relation to the art object, both the artist's and our own, there is an attempt to make good the deficit in human understanding:* 'what I cannot get from the person (originally the mother) in the way of syntonic reflections, I will make for myself through the created object.'" He continues, "The process of creation can be seen as a struggle on two fronts: firstly, to create a medium which is more adaptive and responsive to the artist's need than the mother originally was; secondly, with the help of this medium, as though it were a kind of surrogate mother, to create an object which furthers the realization of the artist's self." (*British Journal of Psychotherapy*, 14(4) (1998) 462, 464.

9. Peter Fuller, *Art and Psychoanalysis* (London: Writers and Readers Cooperative, 1980), p. 175.

10. Jerome D. Oremland, *The Origins and Psychodynamics of Creativity: A Psychoanalytic Perspective*. (Madison, CT: International Universities Press, 1997), p.39. See D.W. Winnicott, *Playing and Reality* (London: Tavistock, 1971), p.112, for a strong evocation of this reciprocity. See also Kenneth Wright, *Vision and Separation between Mother and Baby* (Northvale, NJ: Jason Aronson, 1991), p. 22. Emphasizing the primacy of visual experience, Wright describes the "looking space" where mental representations of attachment may become symbols, pp. 245 f.

11. Daniel N. Stern, *The Interpersonal World of the Infant: A View from Psychoanalysis and Developmental Psychology* (New York: Basic Books, 1985), pp. 21–2; See also T. Berry Brazleton and Michael W. Yogman, "Reciprocity, Attachment and Effectance: Anlage in Early Infancy," *Affective Development in Infancy* (Norwood, NJ: Ablex, 1986) and Caroll E. Izzard, "Facial Expressions and the Regulation of Emotions," *Journal of Personality and Social Psychology*, 58, no. 3 (1990): 487f.

12. Allan N. Schore, *Affect Regulation and the Origin of the Self: The Neurobiology of Emotional Development* (Hillsdale, NJ: Lawrence Erlbaum, 1994), p. 175.

13. Ibid., p. 400f. For a summary of how mother-infant interaction affects the infant's ability to adapt to psycho-physiological stress, see p. 412f. For discussion of how infant-mother miscoordinations invoke 'repair' see Edward Z. Tronick and Jeffery F. Cohn, "Infant-Mother Face-to-Face Interaction: Age and Gender Differences in Coordination and the Occurrence of Miscoordination," *Child Development*, 60 (1989): 85–92.

14. Parker E. Lichtenstein, "Genius as Productive Neurosis," *The Psychological Record*, 21(1971):151–64.

15. Gilbert J. Rose, *The Power of Form: A Psychoanalytic Approach to Aesthetic Form* (Madison, CT: International Universities Press, 1992), p. 226.

16. Gilbert J. Rose, *Necessary Illusion: Art as Witness* (Madison, CT: International Universities Press, 1969), 112. Rose also comments: "Psychoanalysis, through verbalization, undoes repression; art through sensuous forms, counteracts denial. Both restore feeling, or more precisely, awareness of affect to thought and perception, broadening the integrative scope of the ego's reality-testing, and thus contribute to the ongoing mastery of inner and outer reality". *Trauma and Mastery in Life and Art* (New Haven, CT: Yale University Press, 1987), p. xi.

17. Susan Kavaler-Adler, *The Compulsion to Create: A Psychoanalytic Study of Women Artists* (New York: Routledge, 1993), p.11.

18. Ibid., p. 298.

19. Ibid., p.103.For her study of how traumatized female artists become entrapped in self-destructive "demon lover" obsessions see *The Creative Mystique: From Red Shoes Frenzy to Love and Creativity* (New York: Routledge, 1996).

Part I

Central Concepts

1

Anxiety, Adaptation and Fear

I Anxiety and Adaptation

Bowlby's theory of developmental psychodynamics is best termed a psychobiology of the emotions, and his mentor was Charles Darwin. While Darwin's work on emotion remained mainly at the descriptive level in *The Expression of Emotions in Man and Animals* (1872), Bowlby's was a critique and re-description of the early twentieth century depth psychologies he considered to lack grounding in evolutionary theory. Adaptation and survival are thus central concepts for Bowlby, with little room for speculative metapsychologies. Bowlby is interested in the adequacy of emotional control systems within evolved species striving for survival. His focus is on child development in a framework of evolutionary adaptedness. If individuals survive and function well in life, it is because they have genetic endowments to do so and because they have acquired psychodynamic action-systems in the developmental processes. To strengthen this argument, Bowlby draws on the evolutionist Walter Cannon's theory of homeostasis which was first derived from physiological observations. Cannon wrote that "The perfection of the process of holding a stable state in spite of extensive shifts of outer circumstance is not a special gift bestowed upon the highest organisms but is the consequence of a higher evolution".[1] While physiological homeostatic processes may have gained over evolutionary time a high degree of reliability in maintaining safety for individuals, the complex psychological problems of humans introduce challenges homeostatic functions are hard pressed to meet.

Bowlby's theory of normal attachment and its deviations accounts for much human suffering and, in my view, the existence of creativity as a corrective process. Summarizing the work of the physiologist Claude Bernard, Walter Cannon said, "As a rule, whenever conditions are such as to affect the organism harmfully, factors appear within the organism itself that protect it or restore its disturbed balance".[2] Bowlby much preferred Cannon's idea of the balancing function of homeostasis in dynamic psychophysiological imbalances to Freud's idea of "inertia". "As a concept resembling homeostasis, the principle of constancy seems more promising than the principle of inertia", which reduces excitation to zero, Bowlby comments.[3] Both Cannon and Bowlby agree with Claude Bernard who had pointed out that the *milieu interne* "is the product of the organism itself. So long as it is kept uniform, a large number of special devices for maintaining constancy in the workings of the various organs in the body are unnecessary".[4] Studies in evolutionary biology show how most physiological functions are regulated automatically: digestion, breathing, blood flow, etc. and, in emergencies, wound-healing and the regulation of conscious awareness of bodily states by self-monitoring. But the "special devices" mentioned by Cannon, following Bernard, are in addition to automated balancing functions and may include creativity, as a response to anxiety, to be considered here.

The concept of creativity as repair, or psychological retrieval and integration of "lost" affective information about conflicted attachments, follows from Cannon's concept of homeostasis. Yet it introduces a conscious or volitional intent, supplementing the organism's innate tendency to right imbalances. Cannon wrote: "If cells of the bodily organism are injured, or are attacked by disease germs, the fluid matrix at once sets up procedures which are favorable to the restoration of the normal state. The conditions of the organism, therefore, point to the assurance of expert protective and restorative attention . . .".[5] Such attempted restoration of physical health happens mainly outside conscious awareness, but in creativity the innate urge to reach or restore healthy function is assisted by particular conscious techniques. Creativity is nonetheless biologically originated, as Bowlby's insights help us to see.

Anxious attachment is the inevitable precursor of creativity, if Bowlby is correct. He writes that "attachment behaviour ... is the result of the activity of behavioral systems that have a continuing set goal, the specification of which is a certain sort of relationship to another specified individual".[6] If this set goal is frustrated or blocked, a series of reactions, especially in children, may be expected: protest, despair and eventually, detachment.

Examples in which each of these reactions predominates are readily cited in the arts as products of creative efforts at inducing psychological homeostasis. But the principle by which corrective attempts are made have yet to be described. Bowlby gives a further lead by writing: "So long as the required proximity to the attachment figure can be maintained no unpleasant feeling is experienced. When, however, proximity cannot be maintained because either the figure is lost, or some barrier intervened, the consequent searching and striving are accompanied by a sense of disquiet, more or less acute; and the same is true when loss is threatened. In this disquiet at separation and at threat of separation Freud in his later work came to see 'the key to an understanding of anxiety' ".[7] Anxiety as acute disquiet at lost or disturbed attachments is a key issue needing elaboration if the power and persistence of creativity in culture is to make sense. But first it may be asked why Bowlby, and Freud before him, did not make more of Cannon's insistence on innate repair functions linked to those which maintain steady-state physiological functions essential to life.

The answer must be that a continuity is not easily demonstrated; assertions of naturally creative urges are problematic and open to doubt at the more highly elaborated levels in the arts. Once a psychological component is introduced, matters become complicated, and culture itself as a determiner of new creative endeavor has to be reckoned with. To make the argument for creativity as innately adaptive, based on Freud's understanding of anxiety, it is necessary to retrace thinking about physiological repair and regeneration. Using the principle of homeostasis, it may be possible to show a convincing continuity from tissue regeneration and repair at the physiological level to psychological reorganization when the attachment system is disrupted. To preserve itself from dissonance and disorganization, the psyche too may have evolved means to maintain tensions at constant, optimal levels of excitement and attention. What the limits of endurance to insult of the attachment system are within optimal parameters, how likely that insults can be met constructively with lasting good results, and what the restorative means actually may be, are questions to be asked. While the answers are not invariably reassuring, they will point to reassessment of what the creative arts are about considered in a psychobiological frame of reference. If Bowlby's work on attachment seems austere biological fundamentalism, it is because psychodynamic theories emanating from Freud and Melanie Klein lost their power to explain phenomena seen both clinically and in culture. It may be that a new paradigm, designed to promote "steady representational state[s]", can be demonstrated.[8]

II Fear

To understand creativity in adaptive terms, its probable origin in anxiety needs discussion. Anxiety, along with fear and panic, is a life-protecting product of evolution. It is a response to threat in the environment but, unlike fear, it is diffuse and non-specific as to what the danger actually is. Anxiety is both unpleasant and mysterious since its origin is not easily assigned. Psychologists speak of fear mobilizing for the fight or flight which constitutes appropriate action, whereas anxiety is not so easily discharged and is "left in the system". Left in the system, it may diminish rather than enhance its adaptive function, and highly anxious persons may well find themselves more at risk than if the feeling were not so strong, or if it were conscious fear. Panic is obviously a still more maladaptive extreme. The problem, then, is how protective apprehension of danger locks into the emotions as anxiety that cannot be readily transformed into useful information.

"Evolutionary memory" of past danger is a sort of preparedness for risk to life from animal predators and other threats. As a rule, we avoid snakes and dark places, avoidances which may be genetically assisted, but this alone does not explain the array and intensity of anxieties complicating the emotional lives of persons in a society free of snakes and brightly lit. Why so many persons have a low threshold for anxiety-producing stimuli, both internal and external, is not easily explained. More needs to be known about how emotionally relevant events and interactions heighten anxiety rather than lead to fulfilling actions. Threat is subjective, and even the more behaviorist and cognitive theorists admit that "because threatening stimuli are located by automatic perceptual mechanisms, the person is not necessarily aware of the anxiety-eliciting stimulus".[9] In other words, unconscious factors operate in producing anxiety. Blocked fear leaving anxiety in the system, and the possibility of depression, must be considered together.

The question is: how is fear trapped in the system as more generalized anxiety, and what maintains it there? How are low thresholds for arousal of anxiety to be accounted for and what governs helpful or unhelpful pathways of discharge? Bowlby's ethological and human infant studies give guidance with these questions. Differing from Freud and much more from Melanie Klein, Bowlby argues that fear is a natural evolutionary endowment in humans, not to be judged pathological unless by reason of its absence or excess. Fear is adaptive for survival, as may be objectively verified, and we bear evolutionary programs for continuously assessing clues as to levels of safety and danger in which we feel ourselves to be.[10] Fear is a regulator of homeostatic balance in the body-mind complex, and it is increased or reduced according to the rule of homeostasis.[11] In attachment theory, the worst possible stressor, leading to build-up and defensive exclusion of unwanted affect, is being left alone —abandonment without a caretaker especially in infancy and early childhood. Everyone recognizes the fright that comes of abandonment, an obvious source of ongoing apprehension too little recognized in psychoanalysis. So basic to existence is our constant monitoring of safe and unsafe proximity to caregivers, that it is readily forgotten. Also forgotten, or defensively excluded from awareness, is our detailed personal history of alarms, of feeling at risk of not being cared for, of being unwanted or manipulated. As the psychologist Arne Öhman writes, "there appears to be a perceptual system that automatically and preattentively focuses attention on potentially threatening stimuli, in cases where the threat has a likely origin in biological evolution".[12] But whereas Öhman, and other psychologists, only tie fear and anxiety to "expectancy systems" and "memorial representations of past experience" Bowlby proposes an attachment system, beginning with mothers and infants, from which varying developmental pathways open up.

Anxious attachment of some sort may be expected along all sub-optimal developmental pathways where mothers and infants/children are not harmoniously attuned. The programs of expectation written into infants and children determine how subject to anxiety, as opposed to reacting realistically to danger, they are likely to be as adults. Chronic, low threshold anxiety traces more convincingly to feelings of unreliability of maternal attachment than to any other source, according to Bowlby, Ainsworthand their co-workers. To sum up his position, Bowlby writes, "when a child or an adult is afraid of some external object or situation, what he is afraid of is the absence of someone he loves".[13] The most sensitive periods for forming secure attachments are about six months to about five years, when gradual diminishing sensitivity occurs. Patterns of expectation last a lifetime. Modification of these patterns is difficult to introduce, even by creativity, proposed here as means of alleviating anxiety-laden expectations of inter-personal interactions. Thus when assessing the meaning of anxiety disorders, attachment theorists insist upon the study of actual experiences of infants and children, rather than on assumed developmental stages.

It may therefore seem strange that Bowlby's warrant for reassessing basic psychoanalytic assumptions should have been Freud's paper "Inhibitions, Symptoms and Anxiety" (1926). This paper is so remarkable and atypical of Freud that it stands out in his works, explained less as a natural extension of earlier theories of development than as an answer to Otto Rank's challenge that all anxiety arises from birth trauma. Originally believing that anxiety arises from frustrated libido (sexual energy), Freud changed his mind to answer Rank by saying that anxiety arises farther along the continuum: with trauma of separation from mother. As Ernest Jones wrote, looking back on Freud's change of mind, he had seen "a situation of helplessness in which the subject is unable without assistance to master some excessive excitation".[14] That is, alarm at threat of abandonment and ultimate loss of mother was so strong as to overload the system with stimuli which remained internalized as hypersensitivity to renewed threats of loss. In this profound insight, we have the modern origin of attachment theory which, when elaborated in an ethological framework, critiques Freud's entire system, including his 1897 reversal of the trauma theory of neurosis. He evidently did not see or wish to say that his new insights about the origin of anxiety, together with those into depression in "Mourning and Melancholia" (1917), gave trauma a centrality in psychopathology officially denied by psychoanalysis. The lasting implications of this inconsistency reappear throughout discussions of theories of creativity from Klein to Fairbairn, Winnicott, Alice Miller and other revisionists. After years of clinical experience refuting drive theory, so acute had the contradiction become that Bowlby attempted a fundamental revision of psychodynamic theory, whose consequences have yet to be fully appreciated.[15] Bowlby was less interested in showing Freud contradicting himself than in building a new paradigm of mental health starting with primary attachment.

Attachment theory thus gives a first paradigm for redefining human nature and meaning, and Bowlby's formulation invites supplementing and refining. As noted, anxious attachment is a broad concept clarified by Mary Ainsworth's replicable studies showing three attachment categories: secure, anxious-avoidant and anxious-resistant. These require further discussion as to what anxiety actually implies in the latter two categories, and what follows in terms of self-correcting measures. The work of Ainsworth's students: Mary Main on the Adult Attachment Interview; and Patricia Crittenden on classification of attachment styles, and self-maintaining homeostatic systems, will be discussed in the context of innate regenerative urges. Further, Walter Cannon's idea of homeostasis as a series of psycho-physiological regulatory functions has been usefully extended into psychiatry by George L. Engel. Engel not only refined Cannon's fight-flight reactions, he added the concept of "conservation-withdrawal" in discussing depressive reactions as protective for persons in certain adverse circumstances. While fight-flight acts out, conservation-withdrawal acts in—in attempts at self-correcting depressive internalized attachments.[16] Overcoming depressive affect is a major consideration in all theories of creativity, and attachment theory puts new light on the question of what depression actually is and how it is experienced and sometimes relieved. If developmental interpersonal relations strongly influence later depressive moods and "action systems", it must be due to under- or overloading the attachment system . Homeostatically governed corrections suggest enquiry into self-representational symbolizing for reprocessing adverse attachment experiences.

Bowlby himself is clear that persons are more or less well served by homeostatic systems in which emotions play a leading role. He writes: "In the case of each form of homeostasis, an individual is conceived as being born with a strong genetic bias to develop biological systems that, being sensitive to certain types of stimuli, come into action whenever some particular measure deviates from certain set limits and cease action as soon as it is restored within those limits. The theory proposed places maintenance of a steady relationship between organism and familiar environment on a level of biological importance only one step lower than the maintenance of the much better understood physiological steady states".[17]

In *Loss, Sadness and Depression*, examples are given of children in hospital, separated from parents, who devised repetitive games magically to induce the parents' return. These games were clearly created to reduce separation anxiety and to fend off depressive affect.[18] When anxiety reaches intolerable levels, Bowlby explains, defensive exclusion occurs to try to maintain interior balance. Variants of mourning, some of them pathological, occur in very young children who lose parents, and Bowlby points to disordered variants as predisposing to later depression. Affectional relationships necessary to healthy development may be skewed in several ways, and Bowlby has more to say about these than about adaptive, reparative measures. His position is well summarized in *Loss Sadness and Depression*, 216f, and remarks on pp. 229f, 246–248 strongly suggest adaptive modes for increasing information processing to forestall depression. He is on the verge of saying that there is a biological urge to create, to correct and to compensate for, adverse attachment experiences. Such an urge follows directly from adopting homeostasis as a governing concept. Accumulated anxiety simply cannot be left to prey upon the system in which it is internalized; something must be done to improve flexibility of communication within the system where fear of loss of attachment has been defensively excluded only to reappear as anxiety.

But Bowlby does not pursue this line of argument to any extent, leaving it to others to draw conclusions from his basic insights. The possibility of doing so is strongly suggested not only by enlarging upon homeostatic theory but by invoking earlier work by Thomas Hunt Morgan and others on innate regenerative functions in living systems, including those psychologically organized in humans. Indeed in discussing processes of mourning, more or less effective in offsetting risk of depression, Bowlby highlights a major reparative strategy, which may well include symbolic creativity. This is a principal strength of *Attachment and Loss* altogether, as will be kept in mind throughout this discussion. Mourning loss serves to maintain life-sustaining relationships by clearing the system of grief in order to form new attachments. Children mourning a separated or dead parent tend to form attachments to nurses and other caring persons, Bowlby points out; but these attachments are only second best and may portend later emotional difficulties. He gives an example of a child who "sought to recreate with a substitute mother, or potential mother, a version of the relationship . . . with her own mother", and of another who "gave up directing attachment behavior toward the nurses and turned instead to the inanimate teddy".[19] But this is as far as Bowlby's discussion of remedial measures using "created objects" runs, and he takes active issue with more speculative ideas such as D.W. Winnicott's on the role of "transitional objects" in creativity. Whereas Bowlby would probably agree that all aesthetic experience begins with the infant's pleasurable recognition of its mother's face, he is not ready to speculate about the symbolic uses of inanimate objects.[20] Inanimate objects appear to him to be mainly palliative, rather than offering means to discover, project, recombine and reinvent the elements of inner states.

The possibility of enhanced communication within the psychophysiological system of defensively excluded fear and anxiety seems not to have occurred to him, or if it did it seemed beyond empirical testing. By staying within the limits of what could be demonstrated about attachment, Bowlby fulfilled his obligations as a scientist. It is time to extend the theory by suggesting that anxious attachment generates the urge to restore safety by opening new channels of communication within the threatened self, and to convert unpleasant undirected arousal into more manageable feelings, images and ideas. Defensive exclusion of unwanted affect is a probable tactic in situations where threat cannot be overcome but, in the long-term, there are other adaptive strategies, typified by the process of mourning that come into play. Invented stories and configurations of visual imagery draw upon, and move beyond, the process of mourning. Information processing goes on all the time and when symbolic languages are provided, very often distress at loss or faulty attachments is expressed in self-informing coded messages such as dreams, with self-healing potential. Homeostatic function can take many forms, some of them "creative", some psychopathological, and we cannot begin to examine all variants and their implications. It is enough to recognize the possibility that the creative impulse serves healthy homeostasis, and that each creative endeavour arises from a distressed inner state as an attempt to restart the emotional system on a more life-affirming course. Creativity assists inner exploration which, in turn, may realign anxiety and hopelessness with their sources in defective attachments. We will, therefore, examine creativity as the missing term in attachment theory, as Bowlby recognized when he wrote: "Fortunately the human psyche, like human bones, is strongly inclined towards self-healing."[21]

Notes

1. Walter B. Cannon, *The Wisdom of the Body* (New York: W.W. Norton, 1939), p. 23. For discussion and elaboration see Nicholas Mrosovsky,

Rheostasis: The Physiology of Change (New York: Oxford University Press, 1990).

Adaptation at the molecular level was reported by the biologist C.H. Waddington in *Organizers and Genes* (Cambridge University Press, 1947). Waddington described embryological "self- righting", a tendency to rebound in an improved condition from developmental deficit. More recently, DNA repair is becoming understood.

Popular ideas of restoration of homeostatic balance in humans were greatly stimulated by Norman Cousins's *Anatomy of an Illness: Reflections on Healing* (New York: W.W. Norton, 1979). However, René Dubos points out in the introduction that Cousins is really talking about the ancient concept of *vis medicatrix naturae* (the healing power of nature), by which challenges to an organism's health are met by more than homeostatic rebalancing. Spontaneous healing in self-correcting living energy systems results in "a lasting change that makes the organism better adapted to future challenges" (p. 16). This was essentially Waddington's point and it may not be far-fetched to suggest its relevance to artistic creativity at its best.

2. Ibid., p. 287.

3. John Bowlby, *Attachment and Loss*, vol. I, *Attachment* (London: Hogarth Press, 1973), p. 23. For Bowlby's debt to Darwin's idea of biological adaptation see p. 53f.

4. See Cannon, *The Wisdom of the Body*, p. 287.

5. Ibid., p. 319.

6. Bowlby, *Attachment*, p. 140.

7. Ibid., p. 330.

8. John Bowlby, *Attachment and Loss*, vol. II., *Separation, Anxiety and Anger* (London: Hogarth Press, 1973), p. 149. Adaptive flexibility in "representational states" is discussed in terms of Waddington's concept of "homeorhesis", p. 366f.

9. Arne Öhman, "Preferential Preattentive Processing of Threat in Anxiety: Preparedness and Attentional Biases," in *Current*

Controversies in the Anxiety Disorders, ed. R. M. Rapee (New York: The Guilford Press, 1996), p. 262.

10. John Bowlby, *Attachment and Loss*, vol. II, *Separation, Anxiety and Anger* (London: Hogarth Press, 1973), p. 84, pp. 138–39.

11. Ibid., p. 149. See also: *Attachment and Loss*, vol. III, *Loss, Sadness and Depression* (London: Hogarth Press, 1980), p. 55.

12. Öhman, p. 275.

13. Bowlby, *Separation, Anxiety and Anger*, p. 171.

14. Ernest Jones, *The Life and Work of Sigmund Freud*, ed. L. Trilling and S. Marcus (London: Pelican, 1964), p. 577.

15. In *Separation, Anxiety and Anger*, p. 27, Bowlby calls Freud's "Inhibitions, Symptoms and Anxiety" (1926) a "revolutionary late work". See also Appendix I, p. 377f for Freud's early insight into "separation anxiety".

16. William E. Powles, *Human Development and Homeostasis: the Science of Psychiatry* (Madison, CT: International Universities Press, 1992), pp. 202–3; p. 414f. See p.221 for G.E. Vaillant's further work on adaptation.

17. Bowlby, *Separation, Anxiety and Anger*, p. 149.

18. Bowlby, *Loss, Sadness and Depression*, p. llf.

19. Ibid., p. 419. See also *Separation, Anxiety and Anger*, p. 139.

20. Bowlby, *Attachment*, p. 312.

21. John Bowlby, *A Secure Base: Clinical Applications of Attachment Theory* (London: Routledge, 1988), p. 152.

2

The Biology of Regeneration

Regeneration of worn or injured tissues is so pervasive in nature that it must have an analogue in the psychology of higher organisms. Healing processes which exactingly maintain the integrity of body tissues and functions surely extend to mind and emotions through the attachment system, connecting soma to psyche. As a psychophysical developmental theory, attachment gives a comprehensive view of the whole organism's development from infant-mother interdependence at the start of life to the internalized attachment system of the relatively more independent adult. Attachment, in other words, is an adaptive mode in itself, more or less flexible depending on the quality of early interactions in the maturational processes. It seeks balanced, harmonious function within the physical substrate. Regeneration in its entire array from tissue repair to psychological reordering of information under traumatic, or at least suboptimal, developmental conditions, needs considering in a theory of creativity. Regenerative and self-organizing functions, which are strong at the physiological end of the spectrum, are much weaker and harder to describe at the psychological end. Nonetheless, it is plausible to think that a continuity exists and can be demonstrated, with creativity mediating information in the system.

Psychological regeneration—an age-old hope of religion and the arts—may seem weak and nonspecific compared to the extraordinary processes that regrow a newt's severed limb for instance, or the immunological processes that restore health when there is viral illness. Although the psychophysical structures of "mental health" are less observably dependent on organic self-regulation, they are subject to it. Religion and the creative arts assume an innate psychological "righting" propensity, as do the psychotherapies which enlist innate urges to integrated wholeness. Somehow inherent in the psychophysiological organization of persons is a will-to-optimal function which runs the entire range from physical to psychological wellness. It is reasonable to believe that self- organization, maintenance and repair systems are continuous psychological urges to integration, while both are strongly influenced by attachment experience over the course of life.

When an infant develops assumptions about how its mother responds as a caregiver, modified and reinforced through childhood, it stores what may be called an attachment "action system". This set of expectations governs its every move until conflicting experience signals the need for modification. Learning can certainly modify an action system toward a more effective engagement with reality unless there is a severe, traumatic break in relational continuity. In trauma, with loss or severe disruption of expected patterns of attachment, restoration, renewal and regeneration become imperative. Like soma, the psyche is set to meet emergencies. We may also think of a reciprocal interaction between physiological and psychological repair systems, the one limiting or enhancing the other depending on its vigor. Physical and emotional health are obviously interconnected, as study of degenerative disease often shows a "neurotic" component, and physical injury can easily lead to "depression", or vice versa. The extent and effectiveness of repair in each area depends on the severity and nature of insult to the psychophysical systems which interact. Repair of traumatic insult to the integrity of the individual depends on the priming provided by nature and culture, that is on the vigor of a will-to-recovery, variable among individuals, and also on cultural "instructions" about how to control overloadings of anxiety.

Creativity at its best is regenerative, reorganizing experiences of anxious attachments to give them coherent meaning. It works to reconstruct into meaningful narrative or imagery the residues of under- and over-stimulations that threaten the integrity of the personality. Lost anxiety- causing information is recovered for reprocessing into meaningful statements about life beyond one's own subjectivity. Portrayal of an enlarged pattern of family relationships together with feelings about them, clarifies the oppressiveness of anxious-avoidant and anxious-resistant attachments. Accurate recovery of feelings and their reorganization is healing, and it belongs in sequence with physiological repair. It is important for an attachment theory of creativity to include the full range of homeostatic functions and to recognize self-organization as basic to life.

Regeneration thus is a reorganization of life experience for its fullest meaning, making sense of environmental influences as far as they can be recovered into awareness. Whether the reorganized sense of meaning is accurate and effective in assessing external reality—which includes differing assumptive models of reality held by other persons—is never easy to assess. The point is that an organized narrative of experience has been achieved, with a coherence that gives its subject more satisfaction than pain. Anxiety over lost or defective relationships is organized into a meaningful narrative which heals—or begins to heal—the rawness of trauma. This may seem far removed from physical wound healing, and wholesale tissue regeneration, but I wish to say that the processes are continuous in nature, and through all species. At the level of human emotion, where matters are often bafflingly complex, we must advance with caution toward asserting an innate healing capacity observable especially in the creative arts. To demonstrate this capacity for meaningful reorganization of experience in the interest of health, we need to review what is known of wound healing and regeneration of lost functions and parts in organisms less "psychological" than humans. The centrality of organization, its impairment and restoration, will be evident throughout.

Is there full continuity between physiological repair and maintenance of tissues and psychological repair of trauma? If not, what accounts for the difference? The argument will be that there are enough similarities to warrant consideration of all levels of replacement, repair and regeneration, but that at the psychological level restoration and maintenance of homeostatic balances have become so complicated in human evolution that their self-initiated function is seriously in doubt. Even therapist-assisted "repair" through integration of dissonant feelings is problematic, despite the organism's overall urge to achieve healthy function.

Regeneration of damaged or missing tissues, together with restoration to function, is a topic as old as the ancient Greeks. Miraculous replacement of amputated limbs was recorded in the Middle Ages, but only with post-Darwinian biological science has there been study of the potentialities and limitations for regeneration of damaged or lost tissues. Darwin's theory of evolution puts regeneration in a new perspective of species survival within which the individual participates. Effectiveness of tissue repair has a species-wide significance in deciding which individuals recover fastest in a dangerous environment. They and their progeny have selective advantages in competitive food gathering, reproduction, and raising the young. The cumbersome antler-bearing deer, the subject of much research on annual replication of antlers, seems relatively less adapted than predatory tigers, yet sabre-toothed tigers are extinct whereas deer flourish. Could it be that tigers were less adept at recovering from the wounds inflicted by their predator, man? From the evolutionary fate of large animals to the study of cell structure, the biological sciences have reformulated the idea of survival through regeneration.

The biological sciences opened debate about the nature and extent of regenerative capacity in all orders of organisms, and about whether regeneration had been selected for or against over evolutionary time. It was shown that regenerative capabilities vary greatly according to complexity in organisms. Edwin Weller writes: "As the phylogenetic tree is examined, a very definite trend emerges: the more highly organized and complex the organisms becomes, the less likely it is to retain the regenerative capacities of its ancestors. It appears that evolution has selected against regeneration not for it".[1] Lorus and Margery Milne observe that: "the most spectacular feats of regeneration are found among creatures with simple nervous systems or none at all: the earthworms, some sea stars and sea cucumbers, some flatworms and, superlatively, the hydras and sponges"[2]. Some of these organisms can regenerate entirely from a bud, and all can quickly repair massive traumatic damage. While salamanders can fully regenerate an amputated limb, a bird cannot, healing over the stump of a lost leg with scar tissue. Although wound healing is ubiquitous in life, from plants and trees through all sorts of animals to humans, replacement of lost parts is rare. Compensations for loss of appendages or organs are pervasive, but actual replacement by regrowth is limited almost entirely to cold-blooded creatures such as newts and salamanders. Regeneration of amputated salamander limbs has been closely studied revealing an amazing capacity for full replacement of the lost limb through stages resembling original embryological development. The triggering mechanism of epimorphic regeneration is unknown, but a sense of "limbness" in the stump generates in orderly succession, from proximal to distal, bone, muscleand skin such that a fully functional limb is restored. When the wound is by an epithelial apical cap, a regenerative blastema is formed from which arises a duplicate of the original limb structure. A blastema forms at the stump only in the presence of adequate nerve supply, or innervation, which allows mitosis. Although such seemingly miraculous replacement of lost human limbs is hardly to be expected, there is recent evidence that "after amputation, nerve fibers from the stump actually grow new connections—some of which activate brain areas that used to monitor the now absent limb".[3] This previously unknown neuronal growth may be a vestige of a lost limb regenerative capability in humans. It is also observed that there is bone overgrowth after amputation in humans, extending the bone as new histological structure in the stump. Further, when very young children lose part of a finger distal to the last articulation, regrowth is possible. The same happens in mice for reasons that remain mysterious.[4] Post-surgical regeneration of the liver and urinary tract in adult humans is well known, testifying to a residual capacity for replacement of damaged organs. As Richard Goss writes, "mammals apparently possess a latent potential for regeneration that has been secondarily inhibited in some way".[5] Goss speculates that in warm blooded animals, there is "something that happens (or doesn't happen) in the early stages of regeneration when the tendency toward scar formation must be diverted to the pathway of blastema production".[6] We must bear this in mind in thinking about response to psychological trauma in which "scarring" rather than healthy regeneration is the rule. The analogy is suggestive, if not complete, and it will be followed. Compensations for loss of limbs or organs are well established, as when a remaining kidney increases function to compensate for its missing mate. But compensation is not replacement, just as in tissue repair, "a stopgap reaction designed to reestablish continuity of interrupted tissues" is not regeneration.[7] Tissue repair, Goss points out, is universal, while epimorphic regeneration is a luxury which most animals do without, adapting to life by other means after traumatic impairment. As Marco De Vries observes with reference to loss in higher animals of regenerative capacity of body parts, "it appears that Nature is more interested in promoting the evolution of systems as a whole than in regenerating their parts".[8]

Wound healing and certainly regrowth of missing organs, are triumphs of reoganization. Genetic instructions, governed by heritable DNA, direct the embryological differentiation that produces varied forms of life. Each individual within each species has codes for optimal development (although they can be disrupted by deleterious genetic mutations); that is to say each has a built-in instruction manual about how to organize, and stay organized for optimal function. Developmental instructions and those initiating repair in an emergency must be genetically connected. The system "knows" when growth reaches its natural limits, and it also "knows" when tissue regeneration is complete—never too little or too much. These hidden regulators of self-organization are imperfectly understood, but they operate in every bodily system and interact with the psyche to produce and maintain optimal organization. The psyche-soma constantly monitors itself to identify sources of distress or pain in order to remedy them. Of course serious disorganization, such as the disordered cell growth of cancers, may advance without early warning symptoms but when the system of checks and balances is working properly, the body-mind silently purges the system of toxins and dead cells harmful to it, maintaining homeostatic balance of which we are unaware—because it works so well.

Regulation of healthy tissues, and their repair when injured, is presumably within our power to understand. Understanding may improve their function still further if it results in collaboration with them. Unfortunately, psychological maladaptations work against natural healing powers in the body, so that they too must be identified and understood. Nonetheless the somatic healing urge is often powerful enough to surmount emotional suffering and keep up "repairs" despite depression for example. Rupert Sheldrake's theory of morphogenic fields proposes that "a causal influence from previous similar forms" governs the organization and maintenance of living tissues: "a specific morphogenic field is a cause of the specific form taken up by a system" although the first causes are beyond knowing.[9] That Sheldrake's theory of "morphic fields" simply renames Thomas Hunt Morgan's idea of "morphallaxis" will be discussed. If there is anything to this idea, then the organism's urge to reinstate lost or diminished function is powerful indeed. It follows that *vis medicatrix naturae* (the natural powers of healing) are to be respected and assisted in every way possible. Although unable to perform the highest feats of restoration, such as healing severed spinal cords or regrowing lost limbs, the body can nonetheless put itself back together remarkably effectively, even after severe trauma. In Sheldrake's language, it remembers what it was before impairment, and restoration measures proceed in logical sequence until the closest approximation is reached. We will see that remembering is also a central consideration in the psychology of creativity.

This enquiry follows into psychology the idea of organization, disorganization and reorganization. Only a certain amount of disorganization of the early attachment system can occur without concomitant interpersonal difficulties arising later in life. Recent studies by van der Kolk, Judith Herman and others of the lasting effects of childhood trauma reopen the question of primary causality of psychopathology. We will ask what correctives to insults are possible. How much excessive or inconsistent stimulation can a forming human sustain without lasting disadvantage in interpersonal relations? Psychoanalysis has formulated the question in various ways, but only attachment theory, assisted by the new research in trauma, does so in ways consonant with what is known of the biology of healing. But before proceeding with this part of the enquiry, it is useful to review some of the earliest work on the biology of regeneration, that of Thomas Hunt Morgan.

Known primarily as a geneticist, Thomas Hunt Morgan (1866–1945) did impressive early work in the biological of regeneration. By revisiting the work done by Morgan around 1900, a greater appreciation can be gained of the subtle interconnections of regenerative processes, and of their fundamental importance. That few biologists followed Morgan's holistic speculations does not discredit them; most prefer experimentally-based reductionism to his broad questioning of the regenerative capacity of organisms. To accommodate the psychology of regeneration, we too need a broad framework, trusting that it will not be contradicted by microbiology. Morgan's ideas indeed help to give attachment theory a philosophical justification.

Morgan's interest was undoubtedly spurred by Charles Darwin's statement of 1868 that regeneration concerns "Different forms of budding, multiplication by division and restoration of damage and finally development, all these essentially represent the realization of the same capacity . . . All this is part of the same great law".[10] In other words, Darwin saw regeneration as not only reproduction but as primary reparative capability inherent in each organism, including man. The biologist Weissmann, in 1902, gave a different emphasis, holding that regeneration is a special adaptive capacity, not a primary property of living matter. By 1907, Morgan reacted against this view when he said that "The regenerative capacity is a primary property of matter and to its known extent it is already part of the determination of the organic", rather than being an adaptation.[11] More recent views accept that regeneration comprises both reproduction and adaptation.

Morgan's view in 1901 was that: "It seems highly probable that the regenerative process is one of the fundamental attributes of living things, and that we can find no explanation for it as the outcome of the selective agency of the environment. The phenomena of regeneration appear to belong to the general category of growth-phenomena, and as such are characteristic of organisms. Neither regeneration nor growth can be explained, as far as I see, as the result of the usefulness of these attributes to the bodies with which they are indissoluably associated. The fact that the process of regeneration is useful to the organism cannot be made to account for its existence in the organism."[12] While inevitably dispute arose over the adaptive (life-preserving) advantages of wound healing and the regeneration of lost body parts, Morgan's statement still challenges us. He emphasized that not only do impaired organisms transform old material into a new part, but they self-regulate cell growth to restore normal functional relations with surrounding tissues and organs. As Jane Maienschein writes, "Something about the nature of the whole made it possible for the individual to transform material and regulate the characteristics of the whole; Morgan called this process 'morphallaxis'".[13]

Morphallaxis, the participation of the entire organism in regenerating lost or injured parts, is also applicable to the restoration (or in some cases the acquisition for the first time) of psychological integrity, that is integration of feeling arising from disturbing experiences. It implies an aesthetic function of the existing configuration to bring about its completion with a missing element, or elements to compose the whole. Morphallaxis further implies natural self-organization as an explanation of how life is maintained, despite repeated anxiety-causing threats. An artist is required by the composition's incompleteness to complete it on its own terms, not according to what he/she thinks it needs. At a certain point of development an artistic composition "decides" how to organize itself, despite its maker's wishes. It is a mistake to interfere with will-to-wholeness just as the injured body can only be assisted to do its own repairs. Rupert Sheldrake's morphogenic fields are suggested, with creativity in hierarchies inherent in nature. Each organic system has need of creative augmentation to reach its destined completion. The creative arts simulate biological processes by giving incompleteness and disarray harmonious wholeness. While Morgan did not discuss artistic creativity, he prompted thoughts about its origins as a possible extension of morphallaxis, using symbol systems.

Morgan's most important speculations about regeneration that may be generalized to the psychology of creativity appeared in lectures he gave at the Woods Hole Marine Biological Laboratory in Massachusetts in 1898 and 1899. This speculation borders on vitalism which, as a philosophical naturalist, he could not fully justify. Nonetheless, in a most challenging statement Morgan put the problem of how a part can regenerate a new whole, paralleling the action of normal development. Regarding epigenetic response to disruptions of normal function, he wrote: "Something more is included in these phenomena ... than can be explained by simple physical interaction or by chemical influences. The process that takes place suggests that something like an *intelligent process* must be at work—I mean that what we call correlation of the parts seems here to belong rather to the category of phenomena that we call *intelligent*, than to physical and chemical processes. The action seems, however, to be intelligent only so far as concerns the internal relations of the part, i.e., it acts rather as a 'perfecting principle' than as a process of adaptation to external needs".[14]

An intelligent "perfecting principle" that brings order among disordered parts implies a vitalism beyond physics and chemistry that made Morgan uneasy. He could neither explain nor dismiss it, risking credibility as a scientist. He took refuge in the concept of 'form', writing that "It may be that what we call a formative force or a vital force is the property of living things to assume a given form under certain conditions".[15] Other philosophers of biology have continued these speculations, D'Arcy Thompson in *On Growth and Form*, for instance. Thompson writes: "In an organism, great or small, it is not merely the nature of the motions of the living substance which we must interpret in terms of force (according to kinetics) but also the conformation of the organism itself, whose permanence or equilibrium is explained by the interaction and balance of forces, or described in statics." Thompson continues "The living cell is a very complex field of energy, and of energy of many kinds", adding later, "whether we start with liquid or motion at rest, symmetry and uniformity are ultimately attained. The cells draw toward uniformity."[16] More physicalist, and without making vitalistic assumptions, Thompson endorses Morgan's view that form governs regeneration. The development and maintenance of specific organic forms (according to genetic codes, as we now know) is the thrust of life. Why, or ultimately how, this occurs may be beyond science. Morgan knew that "morphallaxis" raised as many problems as it solved. He urged study of as many organic systems as possible, experimenting himself with hydromedusae, earthworms, planarians and frogs where replication of damaged tissue is especially observable. All he could say is that successful healing and regeneration are expressions of molecular structure as it conforms to the integrity of the whole organism. The "perfecting principle" came down to each organism having the power to exert its original organization over disorganization.

In the view of Lancelot Law Whyte, growth, differentiation (and presumably repair) continue in organisms because the organisms are imperfect: "It is only the imperfection of the fit, the difference between organism and environment coupled with the perpetual tendency to improve the fit, that allows the working parts to work and makes them continue to work. Life is a movement toward a condition of perfect fit that can never be realized, while there is still life." Whyte sums up memorably, "Beauty is in the forming power", explaining that, "The supreme beauty is not in the form, but in the forming power. The deepest aesthetic and scientific principle lies in a tendency toward simplicity, order, elegance, form".[17] Symmetry and uniformity are deep in the structure of life, with bilateral symmetry observable especially throughout the animal kingdom. To preserve functional symmetry seems somehow "in the nature of things", but when psychological factors are added, the question of regeneration deepens. Nevertheless, there appears to be continuity between biological tissue repair and psychological urges to integrate recovered information about anxious, and potentially damaging relationships. Soma and psyche interact, and it is reasonable to look further for evidence.

Notes

1. Edwin M. Weller, "Regeneration," in *Biologic Basis of Wound Healing*, ed. Lewis Menaker (New York: Harper & Row, 1975), p. 293.

2. Lorus J. Milne and Margery Milne, *The Ages of Life* (New York: Harcourt, Brace & World, 1968), p. 129.

3. *Psychology Today*, March/April, 1996, p. 11.

4. Richard, J. Goss, "Regeneration Versus Repair," in *Wound Healing: Biochemical & Clinical Aspects*, ed. I. K. Cohen, et al. (Philadelphia: W. B. Saunders, 1992), p. 38.

5. Ibid., p. 28.

6. Ibid., p. 28.

7. Ibid., p. 24, p. 27.

8. Marco J. De Vries, "Healing and the Process of Healing," *Humane Medicine*,1, no. 2 (1985): 57.

9. Rupert Sheldrake, *A New Science of Life: The Hypothesis of Formalist Causation* (London: Granada, 1983), p. 71, p. 93.

10. Quoted in L. V. Polezhaev, *Loss and Restoration of Regenerative Capacity in Tissues and Organs of Animals* (Harvard University Press, 1972), p. 29.

11. Ibid., pp. 29–30.

12. Thomas Hunt Morgan, *Regeneration* (New York: Macmillan, 1901), p. 292.

13. Jane Maienschein, "T. H. Morgan's Regeneration, Epigenesis and (W)holism," in *A History of Regeneration Research* (Cambridge University Press, 1991), ed. Charles E. Dinsmore, p.138. She points out that in *Embryology and Genetics* (1934) Morgan concluded of tissues in regeneration that "The old act as the determiners or organizers of the new, and we can perhaps assume that this is a chemical influence. It is not safe, however, to push such comparisons too far", p. 148. Morgan was careful not to make unwarranted assumptions as he may have done in 1898/9.

14. Ibid., p. 139.

15. Ibid., p. 140.

16. D'Arcy, Thompson, *On Growth and Form* (Cambridge University Press, 1961), p.11, p. 37, p. 106.

17. Lancelot Law Whyte, *Accent on Form: An Anticipation of the Science of Tomorrow* (Westport, CT: Greenwood Press, 1973), pp. 119–120, p. 184, p. 192.

3

Regeneration and Communication

Expressive language and imagery are underestimated in managing anxiety and depression: regenerative urges depend on expressive powers. Biological psychiatry, with its attention almost exclusively to biochemical irregularities neglects the developmental life-experiences to which attachment theory witnesses. To understand regenerative urges, and to assess their cultural meaning, it should be appreciated that suboptimal development (including childhood trauma), leads to chronic anxiety and risk of, or actual depression. If regenerative, reparative and creative urges have so far been left out of theorizing about attachment, it is because the challenges of child neglect and abuse are so urgent but so fraught for society. The communicative arts are all but forgotten amidst controversies about abuse and recovered memory, yet a review of theory shows how central to managing anxiety and depression communicative means actually are.

It is increasingly appreciated that trauma early in child development insults the attachment system, storing up anxieties that can lead to depression. Anxiety and depression have always been linked in psychodynamic theory. Karl Abraham wrote that, "Anxiety and depression are related to each other in the same way as are fear and grief. We fear a coming evil; we grieve over one that has occurred".[1] In other words, while anxiety anticipates insults to bodily and personal integrity, depression is the mood state in which it has happened.

Depression is a kind of ineffectual grieving, and may be thought of, to use Freud's term, as "melancholia" charged with ambivalence toward the lost object.[2] The mood of defeat is sometimes thought of as helplessness and hopelessness, but it can have various intensities and durations with differing outcomes. Theory of depression, along with its companion affective disorder, mania, is controversial, with little agreement among or between psychoanalysts and psychiatrists as to its nature and origins. We will plead for greater recognition of "sensitivity" factors, associated with anxious attachments, which were noted by Bowlby and his associates as important in theorizing child and adult depressions. If, as Freud said in 1926, anxiety is fear of loss of sustaining attachments, then one variety of depression is surely the mood state in which irremediable loss is felt to have occurred. In such a state, communication may be severely impaired, as neurological processes speed up while the rest of the system appears to be shut down. Information is being processed but not effectually communicated. Tension and anxiety are unproductively held within the system, impairing its normal outreach. The system needs re-engaging in social interchange, which can happen only if ambivalent and guilty feelings are cleared. Depression is usually much too serious a condition to expect aesthetic release; yet the author William Styron believed himself saved from suicide by hearing Brahms's "Alto Rhapsody".

Styron had lost his mother at age thirteen and had not successfully mourned her. He spent his "creative" life ruminating and fictionalizing over women and death. He was depressed and alcoholic before the crisis from which the "Alto Rhapsody" rescued him: "I do know that in those last hours before I rescued myself, when I listened to the passage from the 'Alto Rhapsody'— which I'd heard her sing—she had been very much on my mind".[3] The music re-established essential communication, re-animating Styron's central anxiety situation but in a maternal, caring register, enough to produce a relaxation response and healing. By reopening authentic feelings of loss, the music restarted the communication system, enabling movement toward new attachments.

Clear communication, both intrapsychically and interpersonally, is essential to healthy development of personality. No aspect of one's experience of relatedness should lack means of expression in the re-creation of feeling states to recover pleasure or pain. Styron had excluded essential information about his mother's loving care, illustrating Bowlby's point about anxiety situations being protected against by defensive exclusion of unwanted painful information. Short term protection against unpleasant affect may lead to long-term distortions of feeling, to evasions and negations of potential for growth.[4] The compounded complications of depression make retrieval of originating anxieties exceedingly difficult, and to initiate essential communication may require special means as in psychotherapy or art therapy. In the creative artist's case, retrieval of anxiety-laden information is self-induced, and may escape notice unless recognized in theory.

As Bowlby's theory calls for "representational" or "assumptive" models of reality, internalized in the interactive developmental processes, their means of presentation becomes a question. He would agree that any utterance, transitory as in everyday language, or permanent as in writing or the arts, discloses preferences and avoidances in attachments. Culture consists of those considered to be relevant to the collective anxieties of a society. The arts do not specifically "heal"—they open pathways of communication for authentic feeling, enabling persons to take heart and find their personal truths because the artist has discovered an appropriate language of feeling. Of course, artists are seldom explicit about what makes them anxious, but they do convey generalized feeling states that enable others to trust feelings of desire, avoidance, and attachment.

Bowlby makes the important point that depression, and presumably the anxiety accompanying it, may be adaptive, the beginning of health-giving re-organization of neglected or lost information about attachments. The adaptive function of depression depends on strengthening diminished powers of communication: "So long as there is active interchange between ourselves and the external world, either in thought or action, our subjective experience is not one of depression: hope, fear, anger, satisfaction, or any combination of these may be experienced. It is when interchange has ceased that depression occurs, and it continues until such time as new patterns of interchange have become organized toward a new object or goal ...".[5] Creativity and culture are obviously implicated, a fact which needs to be made explicit. How society has dealt historically with loss and mourning is relevant to Bowlby's concern with successful mourning of childhood loss of a parent, or parents. Traditionally led by religion, culture gave meaning to the loss of affectional ties; then the creative arts, and now psychology tries to assist with adjustment to various kinds of loss. Bowlby's attachment theory is an elegantly simple naturalistic demonstration of how emotional health is achieved, distorted, or lost. In the interest of clear demonstration, Bowlby restricted his study to early traumatic loss of parent(s), liability to anxiety and depression being shown where alternative caregiving and mourning were defective.

Subsequent elaborations of his theory, especially by Mary Main who devised the Adult Attachment Interview (AAI), show a much more diverse and subtle range of psychological organization by considering current states of feeling about early attachments. The point here is that encoded feeling states are, by their nature, remote and difficult to recover unless by symbolic representations. Main's work depends on analyzing the subtleties of language. To get at working models of reality, as they help or hinder a life, better means of reading symbolic statements, including fantasy, are needed. Bowlby and his followers orient us as to how to see the question of symbolic representations of anxious states of feeling. They do not give explicit guidance about how to understand all depressions associated with creativity. What, for example, of the manic-depression found in the poets studied here: Robert Lowell, Anne Sexton and Sylvia Plath? The proto-attachment theory of Frieda Fromm-Reichman and May Cohen will be introduced as a possible means of clarifying their creativity. In other words, study of anxious attachment is just beginning, and all new leads must be considered.

Mary Main greatly advances understanding of attachment and anxiety. A former student of Mary Ainsworth, Bowlby's chief research collaborator, Main is an experimental psychologist who extends attachment typology by resourceful observation and experiment. Ainsworth developed the "Strange Situation" technique for ascertaining how a young child had attached to its mother. She discovered three basic types of infant attachment: secure, insecure avoidant and insecure resistant/ambivalent—to which was later added a disorganized/ disoriented category. By observing separations and reunions with a stranger and with mother, Ainsworth established these three modes of attachment, two of them markedly defensive against anxiety experienced in formative relations with the mother and designed to maintain self-organization under stress. Avoidant and resistant defences were seen as the child's techniques devised to maintain safe relations with the child's mother as the only source of protection, despite her unresponsive remoteness or unpredictability in caregiving. In the case of disorganization, there has typically been abuse causing the parent to be feared, leaving no coherent coping strategy.

As Main explains Ainsworth's discovery, each defensive attachment strategy for maintaining self-organization and "proximity to an insecure (dismissing or preoccupied) caregiver" results in an "attentional/ representational state" that is "held in place by anxiety".[6] The concept of representational states, specifically tied to early attachment experiences, and generalized to adult "action systems", has strong implications for the creative arts. If Ainsworth and Main are correct, we may look for evidences of symbolic management of anxiety situations within the verbal and graphic representations of nature and human affairs. How an artist sees and portrays reality is linked to his or her anxiety-tinged version of it—to concern with safe or unsafe proximity to objects and persons, based on actual developmental stressors. Desire, attraction and repulsion can be linked to primary attachment phenomena, if they can be known. It may be that creativity is an inbuilt mechanism for manifesting "representational states" and for giving them greater flexibility than they have as mere defences against anxiety. However transformed these representations are, they may always line up in essentials with the original secure, avoidant, resistant, or disorganized attachment patterns, or with whatever combination has been protectively adopted. The poet or painter gives priority to conflicted subject matter which first of all is his or her own. To follow this line of thought, assurance is needed that there really is continuity between early adaptations to preserve attachment under stress and child and adult personality organization.

Mary Main's inspired invention, the structured Adult-Attachment Interview (AAI), gives strong evidence of continuity between early development and present feeling states about attachment. It assesses use of language as indicating feelings of security of attachment on the principle that lack of clarity of statement betokens unease about the parental attachment being evoked. The subject's current state of mind is assessed by coherence of statement to overall attachment classification which catches the subtleties of adaptation: secure, dismissing of attachment, preoccupied/entangled, unresolved with respect to traumas, and cannot classify. These adult categories correspond to the infant secure, avoidant, resistant/ambivalent and disorganized, but there is no "cannot classify" category for infants. Matches between infant and adult results have been readily obtained and there is increasing experimental evidence of continuity of adaptive means when anxiety has been generated by dyadic control. Developmental pathways are more likely to be continuous than discontinuous, with earliest attachment styles becoming sets of cognitive expectations about relational responses. Anxious insecurity of course has characteristic childhood, adolescent and adult manifestations, while the underlying representational model of what to expect in relationships remains in force.

The AAI's limitations are those of Bowlby's emphasis on the developmental sequelae of unmourned loss, although a wider range of distortions of attachment are captured than those he dealt with in *Attachment and Loss*. Nonetheless, the AAI is especially suited to eliciting feelings of unmourned loss, although it can also uncover gradations of emotional and physical abuse. As psychologists such as Anne Roe and Marvin Eisenstadt have shown, early traumatic loss of a parent may be decisive in initiating later creativity; the AAI should greatly assist in prospective studies. Using this instrument, it should be possible to understand more accurately the role of timing, intensity of reactions and subsequent provision of care following the loss of a parent, and hence of the effectiveness of creativity to manage anxiety.

Scoring of the AAI is according to Grice's maxims of quality (truthfulness), quantity, relation (relevance) and manner (clarity)—with plain, direct speaking about relationships expected in secure persons. Hesitations, lapses, convolutions, embellishments and heightenings of style are all seen as symptomatic and capable of interpretation by categories of anxious attachment: dismissing of attachment, pre-occupied with past attachments unresolved for trauma, and unclassifiable. The ingenious method of translating spontaneous language into categories representing defensive anxiety about the dyadic regulators of parent and child need not be gone into here. When coherence of transcript is scored and a category assigned, it is believed that a subject's unconscious has spoken, or been "surprised" into revealing the individual's basic and irreducible "assumptive model" of how human interaction works.

It may be surprising that working models of reality are relative to past experience, not absolute as persons are apt naively to assume. But once seen as contingent, an avoidant, or pre-occupied person can begin to play with reconstructions and possibilities of altering the model to greater flexibility. The avoidant person will probably be more intensely imaginative, symbolic and obsessively pressured than the person pre-occupied or entangled with early relationships who is likely to be more histrionic and demonstrative in reworked feelings about past experience. Possibilities for the type of art (in differing media) to be produced are yet to be worked out, and expressive possibilities in therapy are just beginning to be appreciated. The AAI is a sort of guided autobiography capable of finding the essence of experience as no standard autobiography can do. Because the interview is interpreted by experts in attachment theory and research, it is also a new departure in psychobiography—with great potential for understanding human motivation. For instance impulses to authoritarian control in charismatic political leaders such as Hitler could be much better understood were AAI scores available. Absolute personal authority could no longer be claimed when it was shown that the state of mind might have been more specifically described.

Attachment styles will be linked to the various diagnostic categories in psychopathology; it is unlikely that any emotional disorder has a background of secure attachment in infancy and childhood. Combinations of loss, trauma and emotional dislocation in the parent-child nexus will emerge as the psychopathologies are studied. In terms of mental health, one of Main's most valuable contributions is the concept of "metacognitive monitoring", a sort of insightful self-awareness of one's own emotional processes which confers flexibility upon the AAI interview. Main and others have used children's drawings of their families and family photos to evoke emotional states. They also use imaginary scenarios of dangerous anxiety-provoking situations to test the quality of feelingful reaction—whether or not there will be a catastrophic or safe outcome indicating the assumptive model of how the interpersonal world works. Traumatized persons are likely to envisage a bad outcome, while the securely attached predict safe delivery from danger. Avoidant children, feigning invulnerability, may be object-dependent, investing more feeling in inanimate toys than in persons. Entangled children are likely to mix much more freely in human affairs and to want to represent dramas in verbal form. Even disorganized children show features of symbolic repair, however misguided, in their attempts to reverse the caregiving relationship upon a frightening parent. Language and imagery are thus differently used according to the felt attachment imperatives arising from differing formative experiences. Versions of creativity are found in each attachment category other than the most pathological. Main's work has untold potential for studying directions of the creative impulse, which is basic to the AAI.

Bowlby's insights into the life-long implications of early attachment have been brilliantly enlarged by Patricia Crittenden. Another former student of Mary Ainsworth, Crittenden extends attachment studies into cognitive psychology and describes the interplay of feeling and thinking according to differing developmental conditions. In doing so she elaborates Main's "disorganized" category and usefully offers a psychopathology of the more severe types of maladaptation that come of neglectful and abusive caretaking. Crittenden reconceptualizes Ainsworth's patterns of attachment to show mental processing of information according to how cognition and affect are employed. Children secure in infancy balance affect and cognition, while the avoidant children defend against affect and rely on cognition, and those ambivalent in infancy use a coercive strategy based on affect. A new paradigm of adaptations to varieties of stressful parenting is offered, and can be found diagrammed in *Attachment Theory* along with a full discussion.[7]

There is some useful congruence between Main's AAI classifications and Crittenden's Patterns of Attachment chart in Figure 1: Crittenden's A 1–2 inhibited personality corresponds approximately to Main's D1–D4 (dismissing of attachment), while Crittenden's B1–2 reserved personality is Main's F1–F2, which are qualified types of secure attachment. Crittenden's B3 comfortable is Main's F3 (secure/autonomous), while B4 reactive corresponds to Main's F4 and F5, in which there was some childhood upset, trauma or separation leaving preoccupation with parental relationships but not severe enough to threaten secure attachment. As these persons' lives are not seriously dislocated by past traumas, their creative impulses, though certainly present, are unlikely to be urgent enough to lead to self-initiated intensive reparative programs. More likely their existential anxieties can be assuaged by society's conventional means offered by religion and the arts.

Self-initiated reparative programs in the arts are generally reserved for the more conflicted personalities appearing among Crittenden's A and C variants, which are classified by Main as D (dismissing and devaluing of attachment) and E (preoccupied with or by early attachments or past experiences). These persons are typically emotionally uneasy in everyday relationships and have histories of developmental insecurities with their parents. Crittenden's contribution is in showing both cognitive (thinking) and affective (feeling) distortions of reality to attend upon developmental attachment experiences. Like Main's, this is pioneer work in its very early stages, and we must be tentative in extrapolating how specifically described anxiously attached persons create, or fail to create, reparative objects in striving for better adaptations in living relationships.

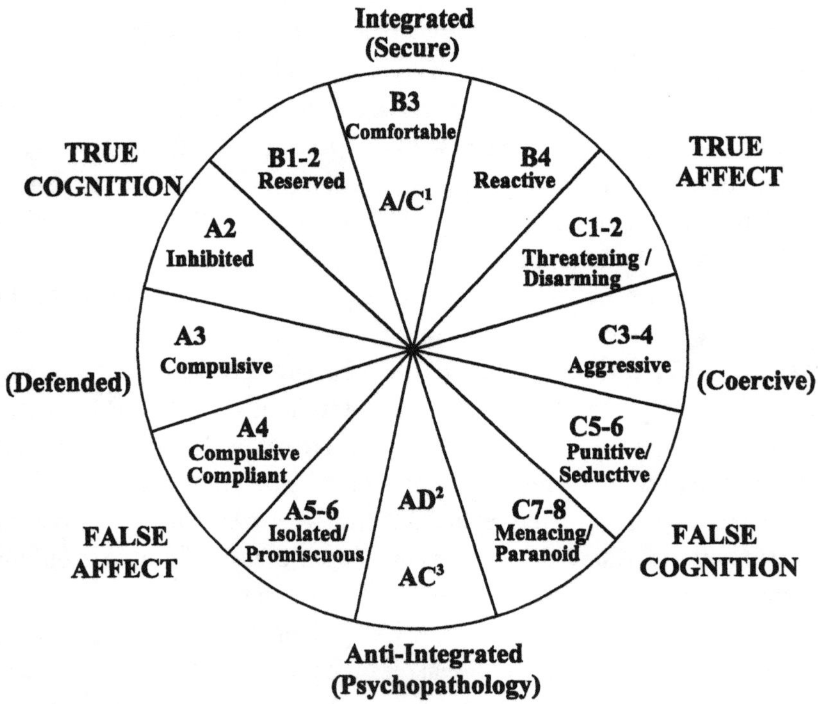

1. Defended/ Coercive; 2. Anxious Depressed;
3. Anti-Integrated AC

Figure 1. Patterns of Adolescent and Adult Attachment, used with permission of Patricia Crittenden

It is possible that some of Crittenden's Cls and C2s, who are threatening and disarming, are also given to spontaneous creativity as they are not so entangled as to be unable to display "true affect" even while tending toward coercive self-protection. Crittenden enlarges on Main's Entangled category with Cl–C6s who are threatening and disarming, aggressive/ helpless and punitive/ seductive; and she continues the "anti-integrated" range with C7 and C8, menacing/ paranoid (false cognition but strong affect), and up the other side of the circle of false cognition and false affect to A5–A6, the isolated/ promiscuous who may be disturbed persons, if not psychopathic. The AC notation shows that there is no integration of avoidant and coercive aspects of affect and cognition, with the "anti-integrated" signifying lack of creativity in these more or less rigidly defended conditions. Each defense strives to offset anxiety and depression, but at varying costs of impaired social interaction and also of imaginative freedom to access the compounded causal anxious attachments. Hostile acting out and blaming others for one's misfortunes is not conducive to the reflectiveness necessary for sustained creative attention to inner reality.

Neither do the A3s, compulsive caregivers, nor the A4s, compulsive compliants, look especially creative as they inhibit true feelings about attachments and act according to the wishes of others. In Main's terms they "dismiss" attachments rather than engage with actual feelings, thus distancing themselves from inner reality. But we should not be too quick to judge and careful observations, together with psychobiographical reconstructions of creative personalities, are needed. Without evidence of artist subjects, the most Crittenden will venture is: "I would expect creativity mostly among A/Cs and some compulsive As (A3, 4, 5, 6) and some obsessive Cs (3-8). The guilty "Don Juans" might be C5–6s (punitive/seductive) [rather] than the affectless A 5–6s who have shame, not entangled guilt".[8] Crittenden's comment on Don Juanism arose in response to an observation that many modern novelists and poets show this tendency.

Crittenden's most promising finding about psychological organization typical of many intellectuals, and presumably of creative persons in western society, is the A/C defensive strategy. The A/C combined, or alternating defence, arises in infancy as adaptive response to mothering that is both abusive and neglectful, or challenging and dangerous to the infant. It is a versatile defence capable of controlling anxiety having more than one focus in the attachment experience. The A, or avoidant component arises from, for example, maternal exasperated withdrawal from a crying infant which increases the infant's distress and sense of danger. As Ainsworth and Main both saw, the result is the infant's defensive isolation of affect and, as Crittenden pointed out, heightened cognitive function as a seemingly safe means of managing interpersonal relations. The C, or coercive and ambivalent, component is affective, rather than cognitive response to unpredictability on the mother's part. Type C infant and childhood expectations are of anger, fear and desire for comfort, all directed toward the same attachment figure, as Crittenden puts it. The urge for integration brings unending struggle, and bi-polar depression is a particular risk for A/C personality organization.[9] The A/C personality may acquire emotional depth by learning to live with life's paradoxes, but he or she is discontent and perpetually disquieted by isolated neediness and wish to control personal relations often beyond what other persons will tolerate. The creative urge for A/Cs fending off depression is to gain access to both the affective and cognitive components of their defences, lest their mistrust fatally weaken their sense of self. When A/Cs gain access to both affective and cognitive components of their makeup, as discomfort and discrepancy motivate them to metacognitive monitoring, creativity may become highly productive for themselves and the culture. Crittenden's insight reinforces the Fromm-Reichman-Cohen theory of manic depression, and it lines up with recent studies of the high incidence of bipolar disorder among creative persons, especially poets. It also suggests support for the theory of "open obsessional" creativity as characteristic of many highly regarded contemporary novelists.

Main's and Crittenden's classifications of adult attachments may seem unduly schematic, even a little inhuman, but they are actually the beginning of a more inclusive understanding of creativity, together with their general utility in theory and therapy. The point about attachment-derived personality organization, with its range of differing assumptive models of reality, is that there can be no such thing as unitary 'creativity', but a plurality of creativities. Each type of creativity occurs within the context of total personality organization, contingent upon assumptions from development as to how relationships operate. Nor can there be a faculty, or even function, simply called 'imagination', as this too is variable according to attachment experiences and defenses against their painful effects. Imaginative function is very different in conditions of early maternal loss from what it is when there has been impingement by an oversolicitous mother. Creating or appropriating images to supplement insufficiency of attachment contrasts sharply with manipulating images to control them. Yet each can contribute to self-organization through creative effort. The many variants in the interplay of defense and creative imagination require observation and historical psychobiographical study. Similarly, fantasy (or phantasy), which differs in avoidant and resistant personality organization, should be reconsidered in a larger attachment theory of imagination. The cultural implications are considerable. Preferred cultural alignments range all the way from the sublimity of traditional high culture to the menace of violent, cultic and pornographic preoccupations depending on emotionally toned models of reality. That the entire range of creative and anti-creative enactments can be related to attachment patterns determined by modes of parenting is a startling thought. It raises questions about how socially approved and disapproved styles of child rearing affect the dominant expressive modes in any culture.

But how well founded in research is such speculation, and how many missing stages are there in the argument from basic attachment patterns to symbolic representations of inner states as in the creative arts? There is little doubt in the minds of ethologists that attachment phenomena are broadly observable in the development of higher primates. Stephen J. Suomi, for instance, reports anxious attachments in Rhesus monkeys separated at six months from their mothers and brought up by peers.[10] Work by Myron J. Hofer shows that "Early, permanent separation of the infant rat from its mother . . . can produce long-term changes in the rat pup's vulnerability to stress later in life" —that is anxiety states.[11] Hofer describes "hidden regulators" operating between mother and infant in the pre-attachment phase of development that articulate with later learning. Hofer discovered ultra-sound communications in young rats, suggesting that such hidden regulation should be looked for in animal and human life as it serves homeostatic security systems. Ever since 1952, when Anne Roe published her pioneering study of the relation of scientific eminence and early loss of parents, the question of loss and creativity has been pursued. Studies by psychoanalysts Mark Kanzer and George Pollock were followed by the large biographical survey of loss and creativity by Marvin Eisenstadt et al., but such work cannot possibly look at the entire life span of its subjects, from infancy to adulthood when creative eminence is noted. Until cradle to grave psychobiographical methods are devised, strict empiricists will remain skeptical about creativity being "caused" by the loss variable.[12] The problem is that of showing continuous developmental pathways, which the AAI with its U category (unresolved mourning) begins to address.

The question of trauma-caused anxiety—including by sexual abuse—later in development may seem easier to address. Persons suffering from post-traumatic stress disorder (PTSD) have had a severe insult to their psycho-physiological integrity, and chronic anxious over-arousal is thereby realistic. It can, however, become disabling when dissociations threaten to take over normal interactions. According to Bessel van der Kolk, "The connection between childhood histories of severe trauma and the emergence of dissociative disorders has become increasingly clear."[13] As van der Kolk points out, many traumatized patients' lives revolve "around repetitive patterns of reliving and warding off traumatic memories, reminders and affects."[14] But he does not connect trauma-caused emotional disorder to attachment patterns as described by Main and Crittenden, let alone suggest how they may be meaningful to the victim and, if possible, realigned. Van der Kolk is indeed aware of Bowlby's basic work on secure attachment, which protects against the worst effects of trauma, but his studies of trauma have not reached a stage of combination with recent developments in attachment research. It is important in understanding encapsulated, inarticulate anxiety originating in, say, sexual abuse before adolescence, and how it fits with earlier secure or insecure types of attachment. Loss of emotional regulation by sensory overloading is complex and not easily attributed to one cause alone. The question of hyperarousal and self-regulation is opened up by van der Kolk, but that of how communicative relief is fostered by therapy is not dealt with.

Marco De Vries's chapter on "Trauma in Cultural Perspective" is more anthropological than cultural in the sense usually meant in studies of creativity. In considering whether culture protects against stress and trauma, De Vries observes that healthy culture is stabilizing, providing groups with homeostatic regulation by meaningful myth and ritual. But when cultures as a whole are traumatized, their health-giving function ceases, as he implies has happened in the West. Lack of any mention of the creative arts as reparative is a signal feature of this discussion. It seems that De Vries discounts the spontaneous urge often found in the creative arts to create meaning out of even the most damaging assaults on personal integrity. For example, the vigorous attempt by writers to understand the Nazi holocaust against European Jews could be cited as evidence of a bold, widely shared reparative wish. Similarly, the psychobiographical attempt to understand the devastating effects of early sexual abuse in, for example, a central writer in our century, Virginia Woolf, gives evidence not only of Woolf's own recreative effort in fiction but of certain critics' wishes to confer larger meaning on her struggles.[15] It is the critics' task to analyze the larger psycho-social context in which such crimes against humanity as The Holocaust and sexual abuse of females can occur. It is indeed the function of healthy culture to reduce levels of collective high anxiety by interpreting them in ways people in general can grasp.

Anxiety aroused by fear of loss of attachment, and depression precipitated by perceived or actual loss, are negative emotional states. When recurrent and severe they spoil normal life and require medical attention, including psychopharmacological therapy. Because drugs often effectively control symptoms, the developmental, interpersonal and intrapsychic meanings of anxiety and depression are easily put aside. In attachment theory anxiety and depression have biological reasons, and are functional states in human survival. Their unpleasantness signals the presence of unprocessed negative information, usually traumatic in origin, which needs to be recovered and reprocessed. Whether called "conservation withdrawal" or simply adaptive responses, unexplored anxiety and depression impede persons psychologically so that reprocessing information, and improved communication of feeling can occur. Anxiety deflects energies to real or imagined risks, while depression reduces responsiveness to external stimuli and draws attention inward to unsolved problems. These are normal responses to endangering or depriving developmental and later, interpersonal attachments. At best, they productively initiate creative recovery of feeling upon which meaning in conferred. This is the point made by Emmy Gut who writes, "In many ways the work of depression is a creative process".[16] When grief, anger and resentment are recovered and processed in a convincing life-narrative, emotional deadlock can be broken. Healing integrative forces can be released, traditionally assisted by religion (contemplation, confession and absolution) and the creative arts which give form and resolution to threatening situations. At best, contemplation and aesthetic awareness promote a relaxation response even in states of utmost threat.[17] With relaxation and associative openness, retrieval and reorganization of lost persecutory information becomes possible. Full narrative competence, gaining access to every shade of feeling about essential attachments, may be utopian but any part of it is gain.

Notes

1. Karl Abraham, "Notes on the Psycho-Analytical Investigation and Treatment of Manic-Depressive Insanity and Allied Conditions (1911)" in *Essential Papers on Depression*, ed. James C. Coyne (New York University Press, 1986), p. 31.

2. Sigmund Freud, "Mourning and Melancholia," in *Essential Papers on Depression*, p. 61.

3. William Styron, *Darkness Visible: A Memoir of Madness* (New York: Random House, 1990), p. 68, p. 81.

4. John Bowlby, *Attachment and Loss* (London: Hogarth Press, 1980), vol. 3, *Loss, Sadness and Depression*, p. 44f, pp. 72–73.

5. Ibid., p. 246.

6. Mary Main, "Recent Studies in Attachment," in *Attachment Theory, Social, Developmental and Clinical Perspectives*, ed. Susan Goldberg, Roy Muir and John Kerr (Hillsdale, N.J.: The Analytic Press, 1995), p. 409.

7. Patricia Crittenden, "Attachment and Psychopathology," in *Attachment Theory*, pp. 398–99.

8. Patricia Crittenden, personal communication.

9. Patricia Crittenden, "Patterns of Attachment and Sexual Behavior: Risk of Dysfunction versus Opportunity for Creative Integration," in *Attachment and Psychopathology* ed. L. Atkinson and K.J. Zucker (New York: Guilford Press, 1997), pp. 83-85.

10. Stephen J. Suomi, "Attachment Theory and Nonhuman Primates," in *Attachment Theory*, p. 196.

11. Myron A. Hofer, "Hidden Regulators in Attachment and Loss," in *Attachment Theory,* p. 219, p. 221.

12. Anne Roe, "A Psychologist Examines Sixty-Four Eminent Scientists," (1952) in *Creativity*, ed. P.E. Vernon (Harmondsworth: Penguin Books, 1970) pp. 43–51. See also: Mark Kanzer, "Writers and the Early Loss of a Parent," *Journal of the Hillside Hospital*, 2, no. 3 (1953): 148–51; George Pollock, "On Mourning, Immortality and Utopia," *Journal of the American Psychoanalytic Association*, 23 (1975): 334–64; Marvin Eisenstadt et al., *Parental Loss and Achievement* (Madison, CT:International Universities Press, 1989).

13. Bessel A. van der Kolk et al., *Traumatic Stress: The Effects of Overwhelming Experience on Mind, Body and Society* (New York: Guilford Press, 1996), p. 66.

14. Ibid., p. 183. See Jennifer J. Freyd, *Betrayal Trauma: The Logic of Forgetting Childhood Abuse* (Harvard University Press, 1996) for "knowledge isolation", p. 15f, and for the first theoretical linking of attachment theory with cognitive changes after sexual abuse. For caution about studies of attachment and trauma see K. S Adam et al., "Attachment Organization and Vulnerability to Loss, Separation and Abuse in Disturbed Adolescents" in *Attachment Theory*, p. 312, p. 329, p. 337.

15. See for example, Louise De Salvo, *Virginia Woolf: The Impact of Childhood Sexual Abuse on Her Life and Work* (Boston: Beacon Press, 1989).

16. Emmy Gut, *Protective and Unprotective Depression: Success or Failure of a Vital Process* (New York Basic Books, 1989), p.202. See

also Crittenden, "Attachment and Pyschopathology" in *Attachment Theory*, pp. 398–99.

17. Herbert Benson, M.D., *The Relaxation Response* (London: Collins, 1976). See especially p. 68f for Dr. Walter R. Hess's experiments in counteracting the fight-flight response with a "tropho-tropic response", promoting restorative processes.

Part II

A Review of Psychoanalytic Theories of Creativity

4

Sigmund Freud and Otto Rank on Creativity

Freud's theory of creativity is not usually associated with his insights in "Inhibitions, Symptoms and Anxiety" (1926), but it should be. Freud's theory of creativity was formulated around the turn of the century and never revisited in the light of later insights about anxiety. His criticism of Otto Rank's idea of "birth trauma" as the source of human anxiety is found in "Inhibitions, Symptoms, and Anxiety", but Freud did not extend his critique to Rank's *Art and Artist* (1932), which is based on the "birth trauma" theory. The present study favours the line of enquiry taken by Rank—that anxiety is the main motivator in creativity—and reconsiders Rank's theory in the light of attachment research. Rank coined the phrase "symbolic adaptation" to the birth trauma, which can equally be applied to "anxious attachment" at any stage of development. Indeed, Rank strongly anticipated attachment theory as elaborated by Bowlby, writing: "the privilege of mutual (conciliatory) protection, social forbearance, and care of others—springs from the natural phase of mother attachment which, on the one hand, rests on the protection given by the mother (womb), on the other, is due to the fear of her caused ultimately by the birth trauma".[1] Anxiety about the maternal function is a crucial insight to follow. Nonetheless, it is well to consider briefly Freud's early studies of creativity to see what may be brought forward from them in formulating a theory closer to Rank's.

Freud's greatest contribution to the study of creativity was psychobiography—however flawed his study of Leonardo and however limited his study of Wilhelm Jensen's *Gradiva* may now appear. In setting himself the problem in the "The Relation of the Poet to Day-Dreaming" (1908) of "how that strange being, the poet, comes by his material", Freud raised new questions about the origin of fantasy.[2] These questions were to be answered differently by Melanie

Klein and her followers, as we shall see, so it is well to be clear how Freud first formulated them. For Freud, childhood fantasy is generated in dramatic play, and mainly has to do with unpleasant experiences: "many things which if they happened in real life could produce no pleasure can nevertheless give enjoyment in a play—many emotions which are essentially painful may become a source of enjoyment to the spectators and hearers of a poet's work".[3] It was Freud's insight that "happy people never make phantasies, only unsatisfied ones. Unsatisfied wishes are the driving power behind phantasies: every separate phantasy contains the fulfilment of a wish, and improves on unsatisfactory reality".[4] In other words, ambitious and erotic wishes arise from neurotic conflict which has origins in unsatisfactory life experiences. Freud is therefore able boldly to propose study of "the connection between the life of the writer and his productions" the beginning of modern psychobiographical studies of creative persons and their products.[5] We need not go into detail as to exactly how Freud thought phantasy/fantasy arose to note that he did not believe, as did Kleinians, that it was innate. It had to do with associations between past experiences and present provocation to realize an unfulfilled wish. While it may be doubted that the writer or artist consciously "disguises" his fantasy and "bribes" his audience with its presentation, it is clear that fantasy arises from transformed anxiety about real experiences. Freud no doubt attributed to artists too much conscious control over their disturbing fantasies, and we now have to come to terms with levels and intensities of anxiety he did not see in 1908. When the painter Paul Klee wrote in his "Creative Credo, 1924": "Each should follow where the pulse of his own heart leads" and "our pounding heart drives us down, deep down to the source of all", we recognize Freud but also acknowledge that such inner discoveries of imagery as Klee's are not "disguised bribes", but authentic communications of strangeness.[6] Nonetheless, Freud was right to emphasize that the pleasure of literature and art "proceeds from the release of tensions in our minds".[7]

There is no hint in "The Relation of the Poet to Day-Dreaming" that "tensions in the mind" might originate in childhood sexual traumas storing up anxiety, or that their release is problematic. Freud had long since changed his mind about the aetiology of hysteria being in the sexual abuse of daughters usually by fathers, and his writings about the arts emphasize Oedipal fantasies in males such as Leonardo and Wilhelm Jensen, where creation of beauty comes of inhibited sexuality. There is a hint of the return of trauma theory in Freud's foreword to Marie Bonaparte's biography of Edgar Allan Poe, where he noted "how that personality derived from intense emotional fixations and painful infantile experiences", but he does not say whether Poe's morbid stories actually released tensions, or merely offered aesthetic consolations for them.[8] There is no denying that Poe was traumatized by parental loss in childhood and by subsequent emotional abuse, but Freud does not speculate about the source of Poe's dreams and fantasies. It remained for Hanna Segal, a Kleinian, to point out the differing content of dreams and day-dreams, the latter being fantasy from defensive splitting and denial, while dreams tell more truth and assist the artist to actually work through his or her troubling experiences.[9] Freud's ultimate views on creativity might be guessed by considering his thoughts about sublimation in "On Narcissism" (1914), for instance. But the purpose here is to show how the creation of aesthetic objects attempts to manage proliferating anxieties with origins in stressful childhood attachments, including traumas. Freud showed that the psychological origin of fantasy can be studied, and he proposed psychobiography as the best means of doing so.

Freud's interaction with his disciple Otto Rank (1884-1939) produced some of the most important ideas about creativity to come out of psychoanalysis. If Freud never revised his theory of creativity in response to Rank's challenge in *Art and Artist* (1932), he did revise his theory of anxiety in response to Rank's assertion that the primary source of anxiety was in the trauma of birth. We will consider Freud's "Inhibitions, Symptoms, and Anxiety" (1926) as the precursor of attachment theory and hence of improved understanding of creativity. But first Rank's reaction against Freud's restrictive account of creativity as inhibited Oedipal sexuality needs review.

Portraying himself as too long "under the spell of the Freudian Idea" of the Oedipus Problem—an ideology he calls it—Rank wished to broaden the discussion of creativity to include fear and will.[10] Rank bravely challenged the mentor to whom he owed his very existence within the psychoanalytic movement, but it may be that he sacrificed too many of Freud's insights in winning a place for his own. By excluding the artist's biography in accounting for creativity, Rank's theory seems retrograde to Freud's. Rank's statement almost contradicts itself: "The mistake in all modern psychological biography lies in its attempt to "explain" the artist's work by his experience, whereas creation can only be made understandable through the inner dynamism of its central problems".[11] How do we know about this "inner dynamism" unless psychobiographically, even in instances such as Michelangelo and Shakespeare where the art so obviously transcends its maker's life?

Rank was critical of Freud's early and incomplete attempts to reconstruct the lives of creative persons according to their displaced Oepidal wishes. He testily remarked that "the whole of analytical pathology has . . . battened on the Oedipus problem", distorting what creativity is all about.[12] For Rank it is the artist's "peculiar reactivity", his creative rather than inhibited neurotic response to complications of family life that is noteworthy. Rightly, Rank emphasized that creativity is an "overcoming", a thrust towards affirmation of life, not primarily a dressing up of hidden disreputable sexual wishes. He writes, "The artistic reaction is thus distinguishable from the neurotic by *overcoming of the trauma* or of the potentiality of inhibition resulting therefrom, no matter whether this is achieved by a single effort or is spread over the whole life-work."[13] For Rank, trauma was mainly birth trauma, and we shall have to enlarge upon his limited idea of fear and anxiety. Nonetheless, when Rank spoke of creativity as "overcoming" trauma, he hit upon its reparative function. While not quite naming it, Rank sketched a theory of creativity as counteracting of fear that rings true and can be developed beyond his insights of 1932. He wrote, "the will-to-form of the artist gives objective expression, in his work, to the soul's tendency to self- externalization, while the aesthetic pleasure of the enjoyer is enabled by his oneness with it to participate in this objectivization immortality".[14]

Rank's remarks in *Art and Artist* are often more searching than conclusive, but they bear close attention, especially the assertion that fear is the prime motivator in creativity. To move beyond Freud's "wish-fulfilment" theory, Rank postulated a "will psychology" in which fear is surmounted by the artist who differs from the neurotic. "I have always regarded the neurotic as a failed artist", he wrote, hoping to show the artist as master of his fears and thus the harbinger of a higher level of self-awareness in society and culture.[15] Rank was so taken with the artist's self-transcending capability that he thought of good psychotherapy as essentially an exercise in eliciting creativity. While genius may be given only to the few, many can use their creative gifts to move beyond neuroticism, Rank believed, thereby freeing himself from the rigid intellectualizations of Freudian psychoanalysis. No doubt Rank expected too much of artists (apart from fragments of his treatment of Anaïs Nin, there is no illustrative case material) but he had redirected enquiry onto highly productive biological lines.

Creative imagination is none other than the inborn human capacity to counteract what Rank called "life fear".[16] By this he meant a strongly felt and pervasive anxiety about life. "Life fear" differed from fright which had an actual referent in impending danger. "Life fear" was a pent-up emotion which compounded itself with insufficient release. Of course Rank had no attachment theory to assist him with the insight that fear and anxiety are developmental risks and may reach intolerable levels in some persons. But he did shift discussion of creativity from anthropological generalizations to individual psychology, specifically to that of fear.

Like Freud, Rank accepts that artistic creativity is a form of play, but not erotic wish-fulfilling play as much as "self-creative" play.[17] The urge to play creatively is motivated by fear of mortality, and while Rank uses the term "dependence", he seems not to have differentiated the ways in which fear arises developmentally, long before thoughts of morality are possible. According to Rank, the artist overcomes "isolating fear socially, by getting society's sanction for his personal immortality-symbolism, whereas the neurotic fails to overcome his mortal fear because he has nothing to compensate it . . . ".[18] Aesthetic immortality is the goal—to leave behind symbolic configurations that speak of self-creation beyond anxiety and fear. Rank did not use the terms angst or anxiety, prime indicators of the modern condition. Yet "life fear" seems intuitively to cover the multitude of anxieties that generated so destructively in inter-war Europe. Indeed, Rank allowed that modern art, ravaged by "the decay of our collective ideologies relative to religion and state", is especially subject to "fear of life and experience"; creativity is reduced to "the biological driving force in the art-form in order to conserve it".[19]

Rank was no doubt wrong entirely to set aside the sexual anxieties seen by Freud, but he was right to increase the range of fears which drive people to both destruction and creation. He was also right to emphasize the "will to externalization", and "progressive concretization" of states that were formerly spiritual or psychological.[20] He concluded, "the will-to-form of the artist gives objective expression, in his work, to the soul's tendency to self-externalization, while the aesthetic pleasure if the enjoyer is enabled, by oneness with it, to participate in this objectivization of immortality".[21] Rank's perceptive statement that creativity is a "biological driving force in the art-form in order to conserve it" gives the most substantial lead to all further theorizing. Rank was certainly capable of analytic realism, yet he knew the value of illusion and would have agreed that the successful art object is an illusionary realm of implied safety and security where fear-inducing dualities are transcended. However, by rejecting psychobiography, Rank left too stark the dichotomy between neurosis and creativity. Further, he forfeited the chance to study more closely the meaning of anxiety producing trauma—beyond "birth trauma". The cumulative psychological sequelae of anxious attachments must be understood before the reparative urge Rank saw makes entire sense.

Rank's brilliant adumbration of a theory of creativity left openings for clarifying and augmenting even in his lifetime. It is strange that assertions about the ultimate source of anxiety, which Rank took from Freud and used in his own book, *The Trauma of Birth* (1923), could have strengthened his account of creativity. So distressed was Freud by Rank's excessive enlargement of his idea of a birth-trauma, that he responded with "Inhibitions, Symptoms and Anxiety". Had they been willing to listen to each other, both Freud and Rank would have strengthened their theories of creativity. But master and pupil were too polarized for successful interchange of ideas.

"Inhibitions, Symptoms and Anxiety" is a vigorous reconsideration of ideas about anxiety by the seventy-year-old Freud . It commends Rank for seeing that "danger situations" form a continuum from the first danger at birth. As implied by Rank, "separation from the mother" is recognized by Freud as posing danger thereafter to the developing child, as implied by Rank. But Freud cannot agree that strong residues from birth traumas cause later neurotic disturbances and that the birth traumas can be abreacted. "Taken literally it implies that the more frequently and the more intensely a neurotic person reproduces the affect of anxiety the more closely will he approach to mental health—an untenable conclusion".[22] Rank's theory "floats in the air instead of being based upon ascertained observations"; he should study actual difficult birth experiences to see whether they produce "infantile apprehensiveness", Freud challenged.[23] Nor had Rank weighed up the effects of sexual dangers occurring later in the developmental processes. Freud denies that Rank's enlarged theory of birth trauma solves the problem of neurosis, but it does contribute to a larger view of neurosis, which Freud goes on to propose.

Improving upon Rank, Freud describes the peculiar human liability to fears: they arise from "the long period of time during which the young of the human species is in a condition of helplessness and dependence" on reliable mothering.[24] The young of other animals have much shorter extra-uterine dependency and are not so liable to the ill-effects of separation and loss of mothers. "The biological factor, then, establishes the earliest situation of danger and creates the need to be loved which will accompany the child through the rest of its life".[25] For the sake of clarity, let us concentrate on Freud's aetiology of fear, excising other elements of his argument about sexuality and the structure of the ego. His insistence on fear and anticipatory anxiety as survival strategies gives them a biological *raison d'être* which psychodynamic thinking continues to elaborate. An adequate theory of creativity is closely allied although Freud does not mention even the possibility.

He might have done so following from the statement that "the ego subjects itself to anxiety as a sort of inoculation, submitting to a slight attack of the illness in order to escape its full strength".[26] Freud had just explained his departure from an earlier view that anxiety was "a general reaction of the ego under conditions of unpleasure",whereas the newer structural view provided for the ego as "the source of anxiety".[27] Thus, taking the ego as the locus of implanted anxiety and as the emotional control centre, Freud could have speculated that it sought to control anxiety by exposing itself to external anxiety-causing stimuli thereby integrating them. Having replaced the sexual "anxiety reaction" with "the anxiety reaction to the *situation of danger* that lay behind it, Freud opened the way to more productive thinking about internalizations of attachment experiences and their attempted management by creativity.[28] Safe aesthetic exposures to "danger situations" could well be adaptively advantageous if this line of thinking is followed. We will show that attachment theory, only implicit in Freud's thinking, makes possible such advance. Neurotic anxiety about expected but unknown danger can be shown to have its most common origin in anxious attachment of the infant/ child to its mother.

Most salutary in Freud's revised theory of anxiety is his insistence that "actual experience" must be the guide to assessing feelings of danger and helplessness. He terms an "actually experienced" condition of helplessness giving rise to anxiety a "traumatic situation". "A danger situation is a recognized, remembered, expected situation of helplessness"—usually traceable to trauma.[29] Freud did not qualify by saying that "danger situations" may also be encoded in the unconscious and operate insidiously out of awareness. In that case, anxiety is difficult to attribute as in "forgotten" sexual abuse, a matter long contentious in his theorizing. Returning to observations in "The Poet and Daydreaming", Freud suggested that childhood "play", changing passivity to activity, helped "to master their experiences psychically".[30] In such a reparative function, he saw justification for Rank's claims about "abreacting" anxiety, though repressed birth trauma is not mentioned. Freud has so fundamentally revised the discussion that the child's entire period of dependency from the birth process onward is an issue, with anxiety-causing trauma potential throughout. The main source of anxiety is "danger of loss" of a caregiving "object"—especially mother; when loss of mother occurs it "is not a danger-situation but a traumatic one", with real pain resulting, Freud writes.[31] He could have continued with a new program for psychobiography and thus for a theory of creativity but, as it was, Freud set an agenda for attachment theorists which is still far from complete.

Freud and Rank were not far apart in their theories of anxiety, but they did not consolidate them, nor did Rank incorporate in *Art and Artist* (1932) Freud's revised theory of anxiety published in 1926. Had Rank done so, his idea of "life fear" would have come out as "life anxiety", a less strong emphasis on real and present danger. It is the diffuse, unspecified sense of risk and menace that is of most interest in the artistic imagery of the modern era; and to investigate it, Freud's aetiology of anxiety in separations and loss is necessary. As Freud challenged, the carrying power of the supposed birth trauma is unknown, but separations and losses are palpable in every human life. Each mother and child undergoes a more or less smooth transition from at-oneness through conditional separation to more or less healthy individuality. To Rank's idea of in-born "life fear", which manifests itself as neurotic inability to face interpersonal challenges, was added "death fear", or concern with inevitable extinction. The polarization of these fears, Rank thought, govern and sometimes tear apart lives. Creativity was the surest way of externalizing these fears and of conferring them in images that supported life and configuring immortality.

But the subtler relational possibilities offered by Freud to explain anxiety leave open the question of creativity. Opinion differs as to just how radical a departure Freud's actually was, and to what extent he started a paradigm shift to attachment theory or only reluctantly foreshadowed it. For example, Charles Spezzano argues that Freud did not contemplate abandoning his non-relational drive and defence model because of any new insights into the causes of anxiety. Indeed, he made little of traumatic separation and loss effects in the ego, a matter of leading importance to such revisionists as Ronald Fairbairn. According to Spezzano, Freud did not mean by separation and loss what Margaret Mahler and John Bowlby meant, seeing them only as an inevitable part of human nature, with anxiety and panic as residual from phylogenetic memory. Proneness to anxiety is as much "a product of inborn endowments of sexual excitement, or of the universal experience of birth excitation having met a constitutionally weak or strong ego, [as] a residue of the joint regulation of excitement, danger, and anxiety by a specifically endowed child and his specific parents".[32] Argument could be indulged around what Freud did or did not think about, for example "castration anxiety" in contrast to "separation anxiety", but here it is enough to say that, following Fairbairn and other objectors to drive theory, Bowlby took Freud to mean that he had, indeed, initiated a paradigm shift to a relational theory of development. Considering Freud's "Inhibitions, Symptoms and Anxiety", and looking also at his *Outline of Psycho-Analysis* (1940), Bowlby said that, "towards the end of his life, Freud was moving towards a formulation not very different from that advanced [in *Attachment and Loss*] ".[33] By working with this assumption, a more convincing account of creativity as anxiety-reduction can be arrived at.

Notes

1. Otto Rank, *The Trauma of Birth* (1923) (New York: Robert Brunner, 1952), p. 90. Rank wrote: "The first reaction after birth is the cry which, by violently abolishing the difficulty of breathing, may presumably relieve a certain amount of anxiety", p. 102. According to Rank, world mythology, and creativity in general, are "sublime attempts to 'undo' the birth trauma, to deny the separation from the mother", p. 105.

2. Sigmund Freud, "The Relation of the Poet to Day-Dreaming," in *Collected Papers*, ed. Joan Riviere (New York: Basic Books, 1957),

vol. 4, p. 173.

3. Ibid., p. 174.

4. Ibid., p. 176. These remarks are clarified in a brief statement on "The Artist as Neurotic", in which the idea of art as sublimation is presented. See *Standard Edition of the Complete Psychological Works of Sigmund Freud*, ed. James Strachey (London: Hogarth Press, 1963), vol. 16 (1916–17), pp. 375–77.

5. Ibid., p.181.

6. Paul Klee, "Creative Credo," in *On Modern Art* (London: Faber, 1948), p. 51.

7. Sigmund Freud, "Poet and Day-Dreaming," p. 183.

8. Sigmund Freud, "Foreword" in Marie Bonaparte, *The Life and Work of Edgar Allen Poe: A Psycho-Analytic Interpretation* (London: Imago Publishing, 1933.) In 1914, Freud had said of the artist, "what he aims at is to awaken in us the same emotional attitude, the same mental constellation as that which in him produced the impetus to create". "The Moses of Michelangelo (1913)" *The Standard Edition*, ed. James Strachey (London: Hogarth Press, 1958), vol. 13 (1913–14), p. 212.

9. Hanna Segal, *Dream, Phantasy, and Art* (London: Tavistock, 1991), p. 109.

10. Otto Rank, *Art and Artist: Creative Urge and Personality Development*. (1932) (New York: W.W.Norton, 1989), p. 63.

11. Ibid., p. 49. See also p. 57.

12. Ibid., p. 63.

13. Ibid., p. 64.

14. Ibid., p.110.

15. Ibid., p. 100.

16. Ibid., p. 101f.

17. Ibid., p. 98.

18. Ibid., p. 101.

19. Ibid., pp. 76–77.

20. Ibid., pp. 102–3.

21. Ibid., p. 110.

22. Sigmund Freud, "Inhibitions, Symptoms and Anxiety," (1926) *The Standard Edition of the Complete Psychological Works of Sigmund Freud*, ed. James Strachey (London: Hogarth Press, 1959), vol. 20 (1925–26), p. 151.

23. Ibid., p. 152.

24. Ibid., p. 154.

25. Ibid., p. 155.

26. Ibid., p. 162.

27. Ibid., p. 161.

28. Ibid., p. 161.

29. Ibid., p. 166–67.

30. Ibid., p. 167.

31. Ibid., p. 169, p. 170.

32. Charles Spezzano, "A Relational Perspective on Anxiety," in *Anxiety as Symptom and Signal*, ed. S.P. Roose and R.A. Glick, (Hillsdale, NJ: The Analytic Press, 1995), pp. 136–37.

33. John Bowlby, *Separation, Anxiety, and Anger*, vol. 2 of *Attachment and Loss*, (London: Hogarth Press, 1973), p. 383.

5

Melanie Klein and Reparation

Arriving in London in 1926 from the continent, where she had trained in psychoanalysis, Melanie Klein (1882–1960) became a highly influential pioneer child analyst. Klein's views on creativity may seem incidental to her theory of child development and therapy, but for decades they shaped thinking about creativity within psychoanalysis, and to some extent that of art criticism, not only in Britain. Always controversial, and at odds with Freud's child analyst daughter, Anna, Klein claimed a special understanding of children by means of Freud's theories. The effect, however, was to depart so far from Freud as to necessitate Klein's own "school", whose intense partisanship brought political upheaval among British psychoanalysts. A nursery school teacher analysed by Freudians Sandor Ferenczi, in Budapest and Karl Abraham, in Berlin, Klein was something of an autodidact, too original to tailor her opinions to orthodoxy and very capable of promulgating them as they evolved.

Klein's theory of infantile "phantasy" was the main reason she aroused so much interest among analysts concerned with the arts and creativity. Freud had stimulated such Surrealist writers as André Breton in France to look to unconscious fantasy for their most powerful material, and an innovative "irrationalism" in art and poetry resulted. Carl Jung opened a line of enquiry into primordial archetypes associated more with adult dream fantasy than with that of infancy and childhood. The arts received a powerful stimulus from Jung, counteracting Freud's narrower Oedipal analysis and showing creativity to be part of humankind's religious endeavor. Klein's program was ostensibly more modest and, while drawing upon both Freud and Rank, it departed into the new territory of child analysis. The overall effect on understanding imaginative phenomena, however, should not be underestimated as Klein's findings in child analysis reverberated back into all of psychoanalysis and its critique of culture.

Without taking direct issue with Freud, Jung or the Surrealists, Klein nevertheless proposed a reassessment of the infant mind so fundamental as to disrupt most presuppositions about creativity. That her dramatic reassessment has proven mainly impossible to substantiate empirically does not change its impact at the time, nor wish away her continuing influence. As Klein's speculations about the origin of "phantasy"changed into dogmas championed by her supporters, polarisations occurred. Two British child analysts in particular, Donald Winnicott and John Bowlby, reacted critically to Klein's basic developmental formulation, and with their reactions altered theories came into view. We should, however, appreciate Klein's contribution before showing that it rests on questionable assumptions about the infant and child psyche.

In this she resembles Otto Rank who also contributed brilliantly to theory of creativity, although from a questionable account of the origin of anxiety. While Freud neglected the earliest infantile sources of anxiety, despite having proposed the idea of "birth trauma" and later acknowledging separation anxiety in infants, his followers quickly made up the deficit. Klein counteracted Rank by proposing that the earliest origin of infantile conflict is in primal destructive fantasies toward the nurturing breast. While scarcely mentioned in her papers, a critique of Rank seems to be going on in that Klein believed anxiety to be innate rather than acquired at birth. She promulgated what her critics see as a psychological version of 'original sin', with its inevitable need for contrition and expiation if 'salvation' is to be possible.

In 1952, Klein wrote: "At the beginning of post-natal life the infant experiences anxiety from internal and external sources. I have for many years held the view that the working of the death instinct within gives rise to the fear of annihilation and that this is the primary cause of persecutory anxiety".[1] Indeed, mentioning Freud but not Rank, Klein nominates the first external source of anxiety as birth itself, and goes on to admit that object relational tensions with the mother do contribute to anxiety in the infant. But concessions to pressures from other analysts to look more for sources of anxiety in mother-infant interaction are kept to a minimum. Klein's papers consist mainly of statements and restatements of how infants allegedly project and introject good (nurturing) and bad (persecuting) breast fantasies. For healthy being to emerge, the latter must be subsumed by the former, though the primal struggle never ceases throughout life. Greed, envy, and destructiveness in children are thus explained by an innate "death wish" that must be transformed and consolidated into moral, responsive behaviour: actual parenting is minimized by this bleak rendering of human nature in which persecutory anxiety in some measure is a given of existence. The saving factor, as Klein puts it, is that "Synthesis between feelings of love and destructive impulses towards one and the same object—the breast—gives rise to depressive anxiety, guilt and the urge to make reparation to the injured loved object, the good breast".[2] By postulating an infantile "paranoid schizoid position" preceding, and to some extent mitigated by, a developmental "depressive position", Klein pathologized infants. Many later child analysts, just as experienced as she, refused to accept this theory which hardened into dogma.

Nonetheless, this bizarre theory of infant psychosis gave rise to a valuable concomitant, reparation to the breast injured in fantasy by the infant's assumed projection of a death wish. Even analysts unable to accept the assumption of a death wish towards the breast knew that sooner or later infants make overtures towards their mothers so as to reciprocate the caring relationship. Even difficult infants do this, so that it is possible to think of a generic reparative impulse to maintain relationship, without postulating a primitive "bad breast" death wish. To be fair, Klein's own words should be quoted: "Reparation in this sense is a wider concept than Freud's concept of "undoing in the obsessional neuroses" and of "reaction formation". For it includes a variety of processes by which the ego feels it undoes harm done in fantasy, restores, preserves and revives objects. The importance of this tendency, bound up as it is with feelings of guilt, also lies in the major contribution it makes to all sublimations, and in this way to mental health".[3] As she also states it, omnipotence decreases in infants as they gain confidence in caretakers. The infant "feels that all the steps in development, all new achievements are giving pleasure to the people around him and that in this way he expresses his love, counterbalances or undoes harm done by his aggressive impulses and makes reparation to his injured loved objects"[4] Elsewhere she puts it most simply: "The experiences of suffering, depression and guilt, linked with greater love for the object, stir up the urge to make reparation".[5] The "object" is, of course, the mother or her breast which takes both good or bad fantasy projections.

The implications of reparation for art are highly important and, with modifications, are more far reaching than Klein's far-fetched metapsychology. Klein writes: "The creative artist makes full use of symbols; and the more they serve to express the conflicts between love and hate, between life and death instincts, the more they approach universal form. He thus condenses the variety of infantile emotions and phantasies which are expressed in them".[6] For Klein, the "good breast" is the primal source of creativeness and, however compromised by greed and envy, the good breast confers reparative powers, not only on artists.

The importance of this theory, and why it appealed to artists and analysts alike, is that it provided a dynamic inner world of the imagination. As Klein wrote in "On Identification" (1955) the "inner world, which can be described in terms of internal relations and happenings, is the product of the infant's own impulses, emotions and phantasies. It is of course profoundly influenced by his good or bad experiences from external sources"—a concession to object relations theorists who were critical of Klein's earlier tendency to seal off hermetically the inner world, which could then communicate only by means of projections and introjections.[7] However pervious or impervious to environmental influences, an inner world of imagination was established as the locus of anxiety-laden contests between love and hate. Klein's version of how the inner world is formed would be disputed by other analysts. Nonetheless, a more dramatic staging for the ravages of anxious attachments could hardly have been devised, whatever her theory of infant and child development. But first, what of Klein's attempts to examine creative behavior?

Regrettably, her central paper on the subject, "Infantile Anxiety-Situations Reflected in a Work of Art and in the Creative Impulse" (1929), is not very convincing. The theory of creativity as reparation to the injured breast needed a stronger argument than Klein produced in response to Freud's recent assertions about anxiety in the paper "Inhibitions, Symptoms, and Anxiety". Klein reacted to Freud's mention of infantile "danger-situations" by urging that they must be considered in terms of the earliest possible "primal scene" anxieties reached only by complete analysis. Such a demand is very limiting in terms of supplying psychobiographical data by which to understand any creative endeavour. Klein was alarmed that Freud should think that in girls "loss of the object is the danger-situation which operates most powerfully"—loss of mother—and in boys, castration threats.[8] Klein's analytic work had proved that both fear of loss of mother and castration fear were modifications of much earlier fears about sadistic attacks by the infant on mother's breast. Such an attack, she asserted, implies the father's penis in the mother, so both parents are implicated in the oral sadistic fantasy. "According to the early sadistic super-ego . . . these united parents are extremely cruel and much dreaded assailants", she wrote.[9] This assertion contra Freud is shrill Kleinian dogma, insufficiently substantiated by her examples from the creative arts.

Instead of using first-hand case material to answer Freud, Klein chose to interpret a newspaper review of a Ravel opera performed in Berlin, together with an article by a writer Klein probably did not know, about a woman painter friend, known only from the report. In other words, Klein made of these materials what she would, and the paper reads like a fabrication. In Colette's libretto for Ravel's opera *The Magic Word*, a sadistic child attacks everything around him, including a squirrel, until the whole world turns against him. Chaos ends only when the child binds the wounded squirrel's paw, uttering the word "Mama". For Klein, the boy's bad behavior was a sadistic attack on his mother's body betokening Oedipal tendencies from the earlier anal stage—to make the point the Oedipal conflict begins very early under "the complete domination of sadism". Klein decided from the report of the opera that the boy's misbehavior was a repetition-compulsion for his earliest persecutory anxiety situation: "The oral frustration which turns the indulgent 'good mother' into the 'bad mother' stimulates his sadism".[10] The "redeeming word", Mama bespeaks the boy's reparative wish. But the opera was only a story, with Klein's psychological assumptions gratuitously added on. Such a demonstration of her thesis is easy to label "wild analysis", or dogmatic capture of a work of art amenable to other interpretations.

The second example in the paper has an improbable too-good-to-be-true quality about it, with no thought that verification was needed. It concerns an article by Karen Michaelis about her friend Ruth Kjar, a depressive who, without training, turned brilliant painter. Titled "The Empty Space", the report is about Kjar spontaneously painting a picture on a wall where a favorite painting had been removed for return to its owner. Made anxious by the empty space on the wall, Kjar's inner emptiness necessitated the creative art—painting the "naked negress". There followed other remarkable paintings by Kjar, especially of family members including one of her mother. Klein explained this woman's remarkable creativity as depressive reparation for guilty anxiety over earlier paranoid projections and the dread of being left alone for having attacked the mother in infantile fantasy. "The little girl has a sadistic desire, originating in the early stages of the Oedipus conflict, to rob the mother's body of its contents, namely the father's penis, faeces, children, and to destroy the mother herself."[11] It was this sort of statement that exasperated other child analysts who needed to know much more in detail about the actual developmental circumstances of depressed persons. It is little wonder that the make-believe quality of Klein's demonstration of motivation to creativity did not, as she intended, enter further thinking. Her defensiveness about Freud's theory of anxiety, together with the flimsy counter examples, lost Klein credibility in the continuing debate.[12] Yet her initiative in discovering creativity as a function of a dynamic inner world of imagination, together with the powerful idea of "reparation"carried forward, as we shall see. Differing estimates of the credibility of Klein's developmental theory clearly show in reformulations of her theory of creativity.

Notes

1. Melanie Klein, "Some Theoretical Conclusions Regarding the Emotional Life of the Infant" (1952) in *Envy and Gratitude and Other Works*, 1946-1963 (New York: Delta, 1977), p. 61.

2. Ibid., p. 65.

3. Melanie Klein, "Psycho-Analytic Play Technique" (1955) in *Envy and Gratitude*, p. 133.

4. Melanie Klein, "Some Theoretical Conclusions Regarding the Emotional Life of the Infant" (1952) in *Envy and Gratitude*, p. 75.

5. Melanie Klein, "Some Reflections on *The Oresteia*" (1963) in *Envy and Gratitude*, p. 279. See also "Love, Guilt and Reparation" (1937) in *Love, Guilt and Reparation and Other Works, 1921-1945* (New

York: Delta, 1977), p. 311; "On Identification" (1955) in *Envy and Gratitude*, p. 143.

6. Melanie Klein, "Some Reflections on *The Oresteia*", p. 299.

7. Melanie Klein, "On Identification", p. 141.

8. Melanie Klein, "Infantile Anxiety Situations Reflected in a Work of Art and in the Creative Impulse" (1929) in *Love, Guilt and Reparation*, p. 213.

9. Ibid., p. 213.

10. Ibid., p. 214.

11. Ibid., p. 217.

12. Attempts to adjust without fundamentally altering Melanie Klein's idea of reparation have not been successful. For example, Janine Chasseguet-Smirgel's "Thoughts on the Concept of Reparation and the Hierarchy of Creative Acts," *International Review of Psycho-Analysis,* 11 (1984): 399–406) usefully distinguishes between artistic creation repairing the subject's ego and, as Klein would have it, the object of projective infantile rage. Chasseguet-Smirgel emphasizes creativity as "self-creation" but, still thinking within Kleinian assumptions, she neglects the traumatic effects of the artist's actual attachments.

Hugh Griffith Clegg's *The Reparative Motif in Child and Adult Therapy* (New York: Jason Aronson, 1984) is explicitly Kleinian, yet it presents a play therapy model which "regards the spontaneous reparative mechanisms as having been inhibited or overwhelmed by some developmental trauma or pattern of traumata. The therapeutic influence consists of allowing the child to readdress the trauma through a regressive recapitulation of the trauma in play" (p. 54). Clegg's valuable study would have been much stronger had it adopted a Bowlby-Winnicott model of development and play.

The best reconsideration and amplification of Melanie Klein's theory of creativity is Hanna Segal's *Dream, Phantasy and Art* (London and New York: Tavistock/ Routledge, 1991). Segal's evident, but unstated, awareness of research by Bowlby and others into the effects of maternal attachment and loss led her to somewhat modify Kleinian theory. Segal writes of creativity as the "attempted resolution of a depressive conflict ... such as to convey both the conflict and the reparative attempt at resolution" (p. 89). The artist's creation of an "inner world" is also, unconsciously "a recreation of a lost world", as in the writing of Marcel Proust (p. 87). Although still invoking Klein's notion of a "depressive position", Segal writes of the actual experience of loss of attachment: "The act of creation at depth has to do with an unconscious memory of a harmonious internal world and the experience of its destruction; that is, the depressive position. The impulse is to recover and recreate this lost world" (p. 94).

Nonetheless, a greater reorientation of theory is called for by Kenneth Wright: "in my view, the primary project of art has little to do with guilt and reparation. I mention this because Kleinian analytic writers, notably Hanna Segal . . . , consider these to be the mainsprings of creativity. To me, what is more important than the need to make reparation *is the quest of the artist to refind, or perhaps discover for the first time, the basic responsiveness and adaptation of the mother* . . . Guilt and reparation may be a part of this process but they are not sufficient motives of the artist's endeavour" ("Deep Calling Unto Deep: Artistic Creativity and the Maternal Object," *British Journal of Psychotherapy*, 14(4) 1998: 459.

6

Ronald Fairbairn: Beyond "Restitution"

Ronald D. Fairbairn (1890–1964) is best known as the Edinburgh psychoanalyst whose *Psychoanalytic Studies of the Personality* (1952) challenged Freudian drive theory and opened the field of "object relations". Trained in psychology and philosophy as well as medicine, Fairbairn's independent pioneering investigations of emotional distress led away from the teachings of Freud and Klein toward an environmentalist theory of psychopathology based on the interactions of mother and infant. Fairbairn boldly and precisely stated his revisionist views which, along with those of Sandor Ferenczi and other Freudian dissidents, have led to research in pre-Oedipal phenomena and successive reformulations of the meaning of mother-infant relationships. Cutting at the very foundations of drive theory, Fairbairn's initiative is prominent in the massive post-Freudian restructuring of psychodynamic theory, especially in Bowlby's attachment theory.

Fairbairn's most succinct statement, "Synopsis of an Object-Relations Theory of the Personality", published in the year of his death, summarizes his view of the dynamic ego, formed by what amounts to internalizations of bad attachments of infant to mother. The mother is both exciting and frustrating, and "the earliest and original form of anxiety as experienced by the child, is separation anxiety".[1] There is no death instinct, and anxiety is entirely the product of stressful interactions of infant and mother, Fairbairn wrote. The greater or lesser intensity of conflict caused within the infant ego by the exciting and frustrating aspects of the maternal/ child relationship causes a degree of splitting into "libidinal" and "anti-libidinal" egos. In other words, the dynamic ego is a system organized and energized by the particular kind of mothering an infant has had. There is no need to postulate a primitive persecutory "paranoid-schizoid position" as Klein had done, but because the ego is inevitably "split", due to some degree of frustration, there is "a basic schizoid position which is more fundamental than the depressive position described by Melanie Klein".[2] Fairbairn's most brilliant clinical and theoretical work was with withdrawn and hopeless schizoid states in the patients who came to him. Fairbairn understood schizoid withdrawal to be defensive against bad early parental internalizations, yet it is also a kind of "creative" solution to distress. But by avoidantly isolating the individual, the schizoid defence proved unhelpful, and therapy was needed to reconnect the isolated inner being to the outer reality, including coming to terms with parenting. Such reconnecting through therapy redirected and enhanced the creative process. This is essentially how Fairbairn initially saw artistic creativity, but without benefit of his mature theory of psychopathology.

From Fairbairn's deliberate reformulation of Melanie Klein's theory of child development (she and Freud are named in the "Synopsis"), it might seem that he wanted nothing to do with her ideas. Yet this had not always been so, both his papers of 1938 on creativity paying tribute to her concept of "reparation" or "restitution" which term he uses in preference to "reparation". As Fairbairn's revolutionary papers critical of Freud's metapsychology, "Schizoid Factors in the Personality" (1940) and "A Revised Psychopathology of the Psychoses and Psychoneuroses" (1941), were still gestating, it is important to see what he was thinking in 1938. Although his selective acceptance of her idea of reparation in a new theory of creativity shows the direction of advance, he never mentions Klein's 1929 paper on "Infantile Anxiety Situations". Both papers suffer from tentativeness as to what Fairbairn's mature theory of human nature is going to be, but they nonetheless are striking contributions to understanding creativity as anxiety reduction.

In "Prolegomena to a Psychology of Art", Fairbairn follows Freud and Klein in postulating the libido as a life principle, coupled with aggression as "a denial of life principle"; he never quite says "death instinct", a Kleinian assumption necessary for her dogma of infantile destructive projections on the "bad breast". While also avoiding the language "good" and "bad" breast, Fairbairn enthusiastically took up the idea that children and adults have destructive fantasies, causing anxiety from which relief is needed. "The co-existence in the individual of these two incompatible groups of impulses inevitably leads to a mental conflict of the most distressing kind", he wrote.[3]

Not yet having arrived at his idea that the ego is object-seeking before it is pleasure-seeking, Fairbairn had little to say in this paper about the interpersonal origin of ambivalence, sadism, and destructive urges. In "The Psychology of Anxiety" (1930), Fairbairn had worked his way through Freud and others to conclude: "The constant presence of a powerful endopsychic menace is certain to lead to situations in which the means of escape are inadequate".[4] Freud's pre-1926 idea of anxiety arising from frustrated libido is all Fairbairn worked with in this paper, greatly limiting its bearing on his later understanding of anxiety states as expressions of interactive failures of infant and mother. By the time of writing "Endopsychic Structure Considered in Terms of Object Relations" (1944), Fairbairn had taken Freud's meaning about separation anxiety in "Inhibitions, Symptoms, and Anxiety", but he does not refer to the paper.[5] Thus the anxious, divided self subject to sadistic fantasies is acknowledged in "Prolegomena", but there is no revised theory to explain it. While Fairbairn had been thinking about repressed fantasies and their constructive release, for instance in "Imagination and Child Development" (c. 1934), he lacked a fuller framework in which to place them.

Fairbairn himself appears not to have been an artist, but he had artist patients, and he possessed an informed sensibility for the traditional arts and architecture. The 1937 Surrealist exhibition in London seems to have jolted him into wondering just what creativity is about. His papers respond to the critic David Gascoyne's claim that Surrealist objects "function symbolically" and Herbert Read's that even the more bizarre manifestations of modernism deserve serious attention. In this historic moment, Fairbairn, the psychoanalyst, attemped to clarify, for himself and a largely uncomprehending public, the meaning of the new art. There is both the shock of unpreparedness for what he was seeing and the awkwardness of a Scottish Calvinist in his remarks, yet Surrealism as symbolic of hidden mental processes fascinated him.

Whereas the leading advocate of Surrealism, André Breton, spoke of throwing off the restrictions of conventional society to embrace Freud and promote all sorts of unreason in dreams and waking life, including madness, Fairbairn spoke only of art being made for "fun". "Fun" is woefully short of the liberation most Surrealists had in mind, Fairbairn's reception of Breton's Surrealist Manifesto (1924) being at best timid, if indeed he had read it. His is a parochial view of a cultural storm that had arisen in Europe and his response to its anarchy was to invoke the moralism implicit in the work of another European, Melanie Klein's theory of reparation. The paintings of Salvador Dali, in particular, left no doubt that destructively sadistic fantasies were on the loose, and had to be explained. Fairbairn's biographer, John D. Sutherland, astutely commented, "Dali's paintings attracted Fairbairn because they depicted the violence of the infant's attacks on his mother's breasts and body along with symbolic restitution".[6] But Fairbairn does less to articulate his fascination with the willingness of Surrealists to reveal unconscious destructive fantasies than he does to show the need for, and means of, their moral containment. He had no inclination to write psychobiography of disturbed childhoods, even had the material been available.

Fairbairn worried over "poverty of art work" in Surrealist painting because of weakness of repression of fantasy, a sign of his faint heartedness in facing almost unprecedented raw imagery.[7] But he did allow that "Art work . . . provides the means of reducing psychical tension in the artist's mind by enabling his repressed urges to obtain some outlet and satisfaction without unduly disturbing his equinimity".[8] And he arrived at an incipiently un-Kleinian explanation: "It is to deal with the anxiety and guilt engendered by destructive fantasies regarding love-objects that repression is originally instituted in childhood; and it is owing to the persistence of such fantasies in the unconscious that it is maintained in adult life".[9] He then developed the Kleinian idea of "restitution" as central to creativity, asserting "that the principle of restitution is the governing principle in art".[10] When a female body is dismembered in a Dali painting, its reassembly, however bizarre, was a morally restitutive act—a tribute to the mother's integrity. In the companion paper, "The Ultimate Basis of Aesthetic Experience", Fairbairn came to a similar conclusion as to the effect of art on the viewer: that unconscious destructive fantasies are elicited and symbolically repaired by the art object. As in the earlier paper, however, he betrayed distaste for extremes of Surrealist imagery, commenting that it causes excessive anxiety, which the viewer's superego cannot tolerate.[11] It is certainly true that Surrealists of the period sometimes believed themselves licensed to produce the most sadistically lurid portrayals of female genitalia, as in André Masson's Freud-inspired "Gradiva" (1939). The seriousness of Freud's study of Wilhelm Jensen's story *Gradiva* (1906) was not helped by such a gratuitous attack on the female body, an attack in which reparation is hard to discern.

It would be interesting to have more examples of the paintings which Fairbairn saw as "restored objects" because they neither under or over symbolized the artist's (and the viewer's) struggle with destructive unconscious fantasy. At this time, Fairbairn worked with a sort of Hegelian dialectic of destructiveness and restitution, thesis and antithesis yielding in some instances the harmonious "restored object", possessing 'beauty'. This highly important conclusion distilled Fairbairn's consideration of Aristotle's theory that tragedy raises pity and fear in order to purge them; but much more it drew on claims of psychoanalysis to be able to heal the divided psyche. It is regrettable that Fairbairn did not rethink his theory of creativity after devising a model of internalized ego constituents representing internalizations of negative infant-mother interactions. Seeing art as a "means of affording the repressed impulses an opportunity for expression and relieving the tension between the repressed impulses and the ego" left the task of saying how the ego was structured.[12] This Fairbairn was about to do brilliantly.

Theories of repression have an interesting history. Henri Ellenberger dates serious concern with emotional "splitting" from a lecture on hysteria given by Jean-Martin Charcot in 1885.[13] In *Studies in Hysteria* (1893–1895), Freud and Breuer developed the idea that hysteria results from the coexistence of two incompatible states of feeling, one conscious, the other unconscious, repressed usually because of forbidden sexual content. The idea of "splitting", basic to psychoanalysis, was subsequently enlarged to include all antithetical, two-part emotional responses, a good accepting and a bad rejecting feeling toward the same "object", usually a person, or relationship, but also inanimate objects. The result is "ambivalence", a term introduced in 1919 by Eugen Bleuler. In "Mourning and Melancholia" (1915), Freud spoke of one part of the ego setting itself up over another, a clear anticipation of Fairbairn's later reconfiguring of Freud's tripartite ego (id, ego, and superego) into an ego consisting of split and internalized contradictory aspects of the mother, the exciting and the inhibiting. Freud's "Mourning and Melancholia" arose from the trauma of World War I, the same war that introduced Fairbairn to shell-shock patients and the emotional complexity of extreme experiences. According to John Sutherland,

Fairbairn's biographer, James Drever's *Instinct in Man* (1917) had convinced Fairbairn that emotions tied to instincts differ depending on whether they are furthered or thwarted, that is, they are invariably bipolar.[14]

Susceptible to Melanie Klein's claim of an inner world of the imagination, Fairbairn remained convinced of a simultaneous split, internalized bipolarity in the feelings of infants toward their mothers, but due to actual relational events. In 1938, with war clouds gathering, Fairbairn still could not see past Klein's idea of restitution to the next stage of evolving theory, but writing on aesthetics perhaps offered reassurance. The harsh reality of World War II pushed Fairbairn to a new level of innovation in psychoanalytic theory—with the full meaning of internalized trauma, or at least, excessive or irregular instinctual stimulation, beginning to come clear.

In 1940, with bombs falling near his Edinburgh house, Fairbairn was still thinking about the arts, but now in terms of schizoid personality features of artists. He wrote, "attraction of literary and artistic activities for individuals with a schizoid propensity is partly due to the fact that these activities provide exhibitionistic means of expression without involving direct social contact".[15] In other words, artists lived in inner worlds of imagination which, he suggested, were built up of frustrated and defensively split negative feelings about mothering with consequent feelings of badness in the self. By showing his paintings or writings, the artist "reveals himself indirectly", "from a distance", which the schizoid personality regards as necessary protection.[16] Nothing is said about "restitution" as Fairbairn envisaged a tough new model of the schizoid ego in which "restitution" would not be easy, or often even possible in his clinical practice. He had seen that internalized feelings of neglect or persecution from bad mothering became structured in the personality and could not be altered by aesthetic means; they might indeed appear to be justified and reinforced.

As Fairbairn continued to focus on an endoscopic structure for the ego, based on actual developmental experiences, the problem of creativity and art receded. His formal writings only once return to it in a review of Ernst Kris's *Psychoanalytic Explorations in Art* (1952). Fairbairn did not much like the book because Kris held too firmly to Freud's idea of "sublimation", which to an object relations theorist, divorced energy from structure. Unlike Kris, Fairbairn did not allow that energy could be discharged by regressions to primary processes and sublimations. Fairbairn agreed with Kris's modest view that his version of a psychoanalysis, at least, could not explain creativity.[17] As this was a book review, Fairbairn did not expand on what his, by then well-formed and clinically-tested, version of endo psychic structure might reveal about creativity.

Had Fairbairn elaborated his view of creativity, he would have had to say that anxiety over internalized persecutory (mother-derived) objects cannot be simply discharged. As the experience of mothering is inevitably split into exciting and inhibitory or rejecting impulses, the ego is bound by this structure. While the exciting object energizes the "libidinal ego"(L.E.) to reach out to new experience, the rejecting object empowers the anti-libidinal ego (anti L.E.; or internal saboteur, as he once termed it) to compromise, diminish or cancel that outreach. This action is mediated by the Central Ego, or moral conscience, little conscious control over impulse and inhibition being allowed for; so in severely schizoid persons, as artists sometimes are, profoundly anxious conditions can persist unmodified even by the most resourceful therapy. In the diagram of endopsychic structure Fairbairn devised, there is no place for restitution but full provision for unending struggle between split, contending, internalized "objects".[18] If an "area of creation" is present, it would have to be between the L.E. and anti-L.E. forces, but Fairbairn's ego has a locked-in claustrophobic feeling, from which only later attachment theory can give release and therefore greater scope for creative activity. The endopsychic predicament as portrayed by Fairbairn has brilliant possibilities for describing say, the moral dialectic in a Shakespeare sonnet, or the bipolar conflict of a play by Samuel Beckett, but it has lost the capacity to speak of symbolic integrative functions, let alone relief of intrapsychic suffering. Fairbairn could no doubt have addressed these matters had he chosen to do so, but he seems to have lost interest, omitting the 1938 papers from his important collection *Psychoanalytic Studies of the Personality* (1952). Nonetheless, however remembered for their faults the early papers on creativity may be, their daring remarks on creativity in the arts as anxiety control should not be forgotten.

Fairbairn's abandonment of the concept of "restitution" or "reparation" was due to more than a general retreat from Kleinianism. Restitution seemed too facile in view of his awesome discovery of schizoid voids in many of his patients. Fairbairn's realization that in schizoid conditions love itself was so feared that withdrawal from human relations was the only protection against intolerable anxiety seems just as dire as Klein's insistence on a death wish at birth, and much more demonstrable. It reminds us of Dante in *The Divine Comedy* looking into the circles of Hell, or Milton in *Paradise Lost* gazing into the chaotic void between Heaven and Hell after the fall and of the existential anxiety both poets recorded on a cosmic scale. But few analysts could accept such far-reaching implications as Fairbairn's, stepping back from the new secular abyss of emptiness with no Christian god to offer redemption.[19]

The most impressive of British analysts who continued to elaborate the idea of reparation are John Rickman and Marion Milner, both strongly influenced by Klein. Of course Klein's followers, such as Hanna Segal, upheld the idea of reparation long after the term had dropped from usage among most other object-relations theorists. Segal wrote in 1991: "What is unique about artistic creativity is that the whole reparative act is in the creation of the symbol".[20] This statement harks back to the brave age when creativity was seen as a positive adjunct to productive psychotherapy, and symbolism regarded (as by Jung, for example) as a means of contacting primordial healing forces.

John Rickman (1891–1951) belonged to the generation of British analysts who had personal contact not only with Freud and Ernest Jones, but with Sandor Ferenczi and Melanie Klein. Rickman's "The Nature of Ugliness and the Creative Impulse" (1940) is an extended commentary on Klein's "Anxiety Situations Reflected in a Work of Art", and it shows Rickman's wartime concern with the forces of destruction, over which he hoped the "creative impulse" might triumph. Rickman took Klein at her word that infantile destructiveness emanating from a "death wish" was the primary source of human ills. It was his hope that the creative arts, which contain the interplay of constructive and destructive tendencies, would contribute to lessening of anxiety and guilt and assist with "a new world built on the ruins of the old".[21] It was a noble vision, but not one able to dispel the fatalism over human nature in Klein's imputed death wish.

Most interesting in Rickman's thinking is his suggestion of a strong reparative wish in persons who see the "ugliness" of the mutilated human form in sculpture. The mutilated Venus de Milo, for example, might induce a fantasy sexual inhibition to be counteracted by the "restorative and creative" impulse. Repressed aggression and destructiveness projected on the sculpture elicit anxiety, which is counteracted by reparative wishes.[22] The entire paper could have been given to elaborating this observation, but Kleinianism took Rickman only so far, and he did not again write on creativity. Overly optimistic though they may have been, the hopes of the early Fairbairn and Rickman for psychological restitution, restoration, or recreation in response to anxiety were capable of more subtle development by subsequent analytic thinkers.

Notes

1. W. Ronald D. Fairbairn, "Synopsis of an Object-Relations Theory of the Personality," *International Journal of Psycho-Analysis*, 44, no. 2 (1963):224–225. Reprinted in *From Instinct to Self; Selected Papers of W. R. D. Fairbairn*, vol. 1, ed. D. E. Scharff and E. F. Birtles (Northvale: Jason Aronson, 1994), pp. 155–56.

   For an appreciation of Fairbairn's insights into schizoid states see James W. Grotstein, "Epilogue: The Fairbairn Legacy," in *Fairbairn and the Origins of Object Relations*, ed. J. S. Grotstein and D. B. Rinsley (New York: Guilford, 1994), p. 319f.

2. Ibid., p. 224.

3. W. R. D. Fairbairn, "Prolegomena to a Psychology of Art," in *From Instinct to Self: Selected Papers of W. R. D. Fairbairn*, vol. 2, ed. E. F. Birtles and D. E. Scharff (Northvale, NJ: Jason Aronson, 1994), p. 388. This paper originally appeared in the *British Journal of Psychology*, 28, part 3 (1938).

4. W. R. D. Fairbairn, "The Psychology of Anxiety" (1930) in *From Instinct to Self*, p. 251.

5. See especially "Endopsychic Structure Considered In Terms of Object-Relationships" (1944) in W. R. D. Fairbairn, *Psychoanalytic Studies of the Personality* (London: Tavistock, 1952), pp. 112–15.

6. John D. Sutherland, *Fairbairn's Journey Into the Interior* (London: Free Association Books, 1989), p. 51.

7. W. R. D. Fairbairn, "Prolegomena to a Psychology of Art", p. 387.

8. Ibid., p. 387.

9. Ibid., p. 388.

10. Ibid., p. 390.

11. W. R. D. Fairbairn, "The Ultimate Basis of Aesthetic Experience," in *From Instinct to Self*, p. 406. This paper originally appeared in *The British Journal of Psychology*, 29, part 2 (1938).

12. W. R. D. Fairbairn, "Prolegomena", p. 393.

13. Henri F. Ellenberger, *The Discovery of the Unconscious* (London: Allen Lane,1970), p. 149.

14. John D. Sutherland, *Fairbairn's Journey*, pp. 27-28.

15. W. R. D. Fairbairn, *Psychoanalytic Studies of the Personality*, p. 16.

16. Ibid., p.19. Grotstein notes "an important incompleteness in Fairbairn's theory of psychic structure: although Fairbairn insisted on 'dynamic structure', he has no image for psychic growth and gives no account of the ongoing interchange which there must be between the central ego and the split-off libidinal and antilibidinal selves. Also, his formulas for cure do not go beyond diminishing the splitting, reconciling the split-off elements of the self, and accepting a more open relationship with the world " (James S. Grotstein, *Fairbairn and the Origins of Object Relations*, pp. 296–97).

17. W. R. D. Fairbairn, "Psychoanalysis and Art," in *From Instinct to Self.* See especially p. 432.

18. W. R. D. Fairbairn, "Endopsychic Structure Considered in Terms of Object-Relationships," in *Psychoanalytic Studies of the Personality*, p. 105. As James Grotstein points out, Fairbairn's structural theory of ego formation is especially accommodating to newer work on the effects of childhood trauma, such as that of Bessel van der Kolk

(Grotstein, *Fairbairn and the Origins of Object Relations*, p. 182).

19. Fairbairn's principal interpreter, Harry Guntrip, allows the theory of reparation but does not develop it in the context of creativity. See *Schizoid Phenomena, Object-Relations and the Self* (London, Hogarth, 1968), p. 387.

20. Hanna Segal, *Dream, Phantasy and Art* (London: Tavistock, 1991), p. 95. The differences among what Freud, Jung and later Ernest Jones said about symbolism are beyond the scope of this discussion.

21. John Rickman, "On the Nature of Ugliness and the Creative Impulse," *International Journal of Psycho-Analysis*, 21, part 1 (1940): 308.

22. Ibid., p. 298.

7

D. W. Winnicott as Tiresias

Fairbairn proposed his ideas about creativity at the beginning of his writing career, while Donald Winnicott waited until toward the end. *Playing and Reality* published in 1971, the year of his death, summarizes many themes developed throughout Winnicott's long career as a pioneer child analyst. A need to understand imagination became ever more insistent as Winnicott worked out his principles and techniques of child therapy. As early as 1931, he had written :"The importance of the feelings of early years can be proved in the case of any one individual in the course of psychoanalyses, and is illustrated . . . in all forms of art, in folk lore and in religions".[1] By the 1950s and '60s, it became possible to write about the origins of creativity in a series of brief, exploratory essays laden with potential for further elaboration. The stated purpose was a corrective: "Cultural experience has not found its true place in the theory used by analysts in their work and in their thinking".[2] His purpose was to elaborate "Transitional Objects and Transitional Phenomena" (1951), showing that the infant's use of a "transitional object" (a blanket or a toy, secondary to the maternal breast) involved a paradox which had to be maintained and could not be escaped. This brilliant paper makes Winnicott's most lasting contribution to theory of creativity, but he could not possibly either fully explore cultural experience or fully relate it to psychoanalytic theory and therapy. The project was too large, Winnicott's experience of the arts too limited, and his personal involvement in the questions he sets more complicated than meets the eye.

If Winnicott's speculations about creativity were aimed solely at fellow analysts to broaden thinking, their limitations would not be so serious. But they have gone far and wide in the world of art and criticism, without full appreciation of what they imply. By highlighting the capacity for mere "play", at the expense of moral and interpersonal concerns that also go into creativity, Winnicott risks trivializing creativity altogether. By weighting adult creativity toward the infant and child's propensity to "play" in a transitional space between itself and the maternal breast, he restricts what is likely to be said about the achievements of mature art. Possibly this is because of his own limited experience of the history and criticism of art and literature. While Winnicott had access to Bloomsbury writers and painters through his first analyst James Strachey, and their colleague in psychoanalysis Adrian Stephen (brother of Virginia Woolf), it is not clear that Winnicott was seriously reading and looking at their work. Through his lifelong friend, the art collector H. S. Ede, Winnicott had many contacts with performing and creative artists; but these encounters seem to have been transient. In one instance, at least, they led to treating a poet.[3] Winnicott certainly loved serious poetry, Wordsworth's being mentioned by friends, but especially he loved Edward Lear's whimsical "The Owl and the Pussycat", which he memorized—an indication that "play" could easily overtake seriousness.[4]

Winnicott lacked patience for the sustained attention demanded by great art. He is unlikely to have given the hours necessary, for instance, to reading Milton's epic *Paradise Lost*, or to appreciating the profundities of Rembrandt's paintings in the National Gallery. It is true that he took Bach and late Beethoven seriously and collected their music. He played the piano well at every opportunity. Yet he uncritically greeted the Beatles and wanted to write a musical comedy. There is something in this of the rebel against Methodist strictness from his childhood, as there was in Calvinist Fairbairn claiming that art was made "for fun". Any real engagement with art, literature or music must be admitted to be arduous and demanding, evidencing that the artist's work had not been much fun, and that engaging with it may not be fun either. Apart from pungent remarks on the contemporary painter Francis Bacon's portraits "painfully striving towards being seen, which is the basis of creative looking", Winnicott has little to illustrate his theories, other than case material and some remarks on Hamlet.[5] He does not penetrate Bacon's dominant relational anxieties, writing "I know nothing of this artist's private life".[6]

Surprisingly, while Winnicott liked the biographies of creative people, he said: "I only read them until they reach the age of four or five—after that they become too boring".[7] But imagine reading about the English Civil War activist poet, John Milton, until he was only four or five, or about Rembrandt before training as a painter. The limitation of this appears not to have occurred to Winnicott, and thus the developmentalist orientation to art is absent. Creativity was a 'universal' about being alive, and it seemed unlikely that anyone would ever want to explain the creative impulse.[8] The result was to leave Winnicott incurious about psychobiography as an attempt to reconstruct the necessity for creativity over an artist's entire lifetime. He could assert that the artist's "finished creation never heals the underlying sense of self" without considering psychobiographically any artist's life and creative endeavour. However sound a generalization, he made no attempt to prove the case. (Freud had spoken of the child's wish-fulfilling play, but his psychobiographies of artists, although flawed, took into account many more factors.) Did Milton end up deficient in sense of self; did Rembrandt? What special criteria would a psychoanalyst bring to deciding and, when all was said, would we have a better appreciation of the art? A psychobiographical question about the painter Francis Bacon's anxious homosexuality could have been raised, but it was not. As Adam Philips notes, although Winnicott thought artists' "drive for authenticity" highly important, he made the qualification for them, and for himself that, added to the wish to reveal themselves, is the "still more urgent need not to be found".[9]

"Not to Be Found" is disconcerting as it makes difficult not only the psychobiography of artists, but also close analysis of artists' works, for instance in the criticism of Peter Fuller. Fuller applies Winnicott's idea to improved understanding of actual artists' works. He notes, for instance, that while it may be trivial to call Cézanne's apples breast-like, it is highly important "that the kind of space which Cézanne constructs, with its ambivalences between concepts and perceptions, is in some way related to the way in which the infant relates itself to the breast . . . "[10]. Fuller draws no psychobiographical conclusions, but he is on their track. Winnicott made no such attempt at applying his insights, let alone at trying a sustained analysis of any artist at "play", or the resulting work. Winnicott the child therapist, who brilliantly invented the spontaneous "squiggle game" to tap the child's unconscious, was an intuitive adult playmate. He was a sort of therapeutic performance artist, playing on the floor, or with a spatula to get reactions while a mother held her baby. Winnicott had a genius at inventing such tactics but, if an artist at all, he was an *artiste manqué,* an antic (manic) doodler and versifier, not a draftsman, poet, or even musician. These are reasons not to look for much support in Winnicott's theorizing for the Kleinian idea of reparation, or for much interest in its reformulation.

A reparative urge presupposes unmastered anxiety for which an origin must be proposed. As we have seen in Melanie Klein's view, infantile anxiety was about a death wish projected on the maternal breast, to which she later added primal envy of the breast. Knowing that he needed to study pre-Oedipal sources of pathology, Winnicott first became a protegé of Klein but, becoming dissatisfied with her lack of attention to infants' environments, their actual relations with their mothers, he worked his way to independence.[11] While Winnicott thought Klein's early contributions to child analysis outstanding, he found them increasingly dogmatic, stated in a "dead language" by her followers. In letters, he pleaded with Klein for a freeing up of her concepts and language so that corrective discussion could make them more plausible.[12] Winnicott dismissed the hypothetical infantile "paranoid schizoid position" as unreal and thought "depressive position" a bad term which pathologized infants to protect their mothers; he replaced it with "stage of concern", which is when the infant begins to regard its mother as a real person with feelings of her own.

In his diplomatically worded "A Personal View of the Kleinian Contribution" (1962), Winnicott wrote that the idea of restitution and reparation, offsetting destructive impulses whatever their origin, "is Klein's most important contribution, in my opinion, and I think it ranks with Freud's concept of the Oedipus complex".[13] But when it came to "Creativity and Its Origins" (1971) Winnicott saw limitations in "the concept of reparation and restitution". While agreeing with Klein that babies have destructive impulses, and that fusion of erotic and destructive impulses are a sign of health, he objected that "Klein's important work does not reach to the subject of creativity itself and therefore it could easily have the effect of further obscuring the main issue".[14] Winnicott was thinking of statements in her last theoretical work *Envy and Gratitude* (1957), in which Klein introduced the concept of primal envy of the breast, a concept he could not accept. There is no reference back to her "Infantile Anxiety-Situations Reflected in a Work of Art and in the Creative Impulse" (1929), nor does he refer to "Some Reflections on *The Oresteia*"(1963), where Klein proposed unexceptionably that, "The creative artist makes full use of symbols; and the more they serve to express the conflicts between love and hate, between destructiveness and reparation, between life and death instincts, the more they approach universal form"[15]

Winnicott replaced "reparative" functions in creativity with "transitional" phenomena, which respected the environmental features of mother-infant exchanges in the "maturation processes". Instead of reparation, Winnicott spoke of "mending" a distressing gap between infant and breast. By dismissing death instinct causality, he perhaps needlessly eliminated reparative impulses, opting for "acceptance of a paradox", but the nature of the paradox is none too clear without further examination of Winnicott's personal view of anxiety.[16] This is tricky as there is little evidence to go on from Winnicott's own childhood other than an aggressive doll-destroying incident narrated by his wife, Clare Winnicott. For Winnicott, creativity was linked to aggression against transitional objects—attack which they survived. In the words of Clare Winnicott: "For him, the destroying of the object in unconscious fantasy is like a cleansing process, which facilitates again and again the discovery of the object anew. It is a process of purification and renewal."[17]

The doll referred to was called Rosie, a sort of transitional object, and Winnicott recalled that at three years of age "I bashed flat the nose of the wax doll that belonged to my sisters and that had become a source of irritation because it was over that doll that my father used to tease me".[18] The attack on the doll was a deliberate act of destruction " and much of my life has been founded on the undoubted fact that I actually did this deed, not merely wished and planned it". His good-tempered father remodelled ("mended") the face, returning the doll to normal: "This early demonstration of the restitutive and reparative act certainly made an impression on me . . . " and, one might expect the reparative act to have been thereby validated.[19] But it was performed by Winnicott's father, not himself; Winnicott's aggression was against a symbolic female associated with his dominatingly female household, perhaps his mother and nanny more than his older sisters. As Winnicott explained, "in a sense I was an only child with multiple mothers and with a father extremely preoccupied in my younger years . . . ".[20] His own transitional object was another doll called Lily, belonging to his younger sister, and Winnicott was very distressed when it fell and broke", after which he "hated all dolls".[21] Winnicott did not associate the bad things that happened to Rosie and Lily with specific anxious and guilty feelings about his mother, nanny and sisters ("multiple mothers"), but such feelings may be inferred.

While Winnicott's upper middle class Devon childhood was privileged and stable, with no conspicuous losses, there is evidence that his mother was sometimes depressed. A poem called "The Tree", written when Winnicott was sixty-seven, speaks of Elizabeth Winnicott "weeping" and of his wish "to cure her inward death".[22] In Brett Kahr's reconstruction of the situation, Winnicott's overbusy father delegated his son to raise the mood of his depressed wife and, oppressed by the task, Winnicott was left anxious and guilty. He was also left with an abiding wish to help distressed women (rescue fantasies): "Analysis is my chosen job, the way I will best deal with my own guilt, the way I can express myself in a constructive way", he wrote in 1949.[23] Unmentioned is the aggression and hostility Winnicott inevitably felt toward the females in his childhood ambit—as symbolically expressed in an attack upon and an accident to dolls. In a sense, the dolls "survived" attacks as do mothers and analysts with difficult patients. The hostile wish to retaliate against female domination, together with its contrary, the wish to repair or mend damage and expiate guilt, became Winnicott's "paradox". While false self organization is compliant and ingratiatingly "reparative", the suppressed "true self" needs to acknowledge hostile feelings and integrate them, not just live by a fragile reaction formation. This is the paradox of the classic obsessional defence which, as Fairbairn said, internalizes both accepting and rejecting objects (split feature of mothering) which remain forever contentiously polarized in the self. In other words, reparative impulses are inevitably followed by another impulse to attack, with no final reconciliation possible, the main hope being that the attacked object (internalized persecutory mother figure) survives. This appears to have been Winnicott's basic "anxiety situation", to which was added ambiguity about gender.

Winnicott had much to say throughout his career about anxiety, especially in the earliest stages of development, but he did not include "anxiety situations" in his theory of creativity. This I believe to be its major limitation and the reason why Winnicott did not distinguish between creative living and the special types of creativity found in the arts. In "Ego Integration in Child Development" (1962), which contains his famous conundrum about the beginning of the infant ego being a "summation of beginnings", Winnicott also made his clearest statement about anxiety. When there is not "good enough mothering", ego maturation cannot get properly started and undergoes distortion. The baby is to be thought of "as an immature being who is all the time on the brink of unthinkable anxiety".[24] To allay anxiety and integrate its ego, the baby needs reliable "holding" in a secure environment—a matter of the mother's style of attachment to which John Bowlby turned with greater precision. If the infant lacked secure "holding" and became confused about its "objects", Winnicott saw two pathological possibilities: schizoid withdrawal, or detachment and self-holding. Self-holding meant development of a false defensive caretaker self "designed to hide and protect this core of the self".[25] He added that anxiety tends to mature into guilt about aggression and fears of annihilation.[26]

Yet there is nothing about overcoming anxiety and guilt in Winnicott's account of creative play. Play is simply a 'universal' that promotes healthy growth of the personality; it is not said to unlock hidden resources of anxiety and guilt which imperil the "true self".[27] Winnicott seems to have regarded the deepest instinctual anxiety and guilt to be unreachable, unless in the most favourable analytic transference. Production of fantasy by artists would not do it, and he emphasized the useless circularity of much fantasy.[28] He went so far as to say that the artist "is able to reach to a kind of socialization which obviates the need for guilt-feeling and the associated reparative and restitutive activity that forms the basis for ordinary constructive work. The creative artist or thinker may, in fact fail to understand, or even may despise, the feelings of concern that motivate a less creative person; and of artists it may be said that some have no capacity for guilt and yet achieve a socialization through their exceptional talent".[29] This is an astonishing generalization, given no further discussion and without examples. What artists was Winnicott thinking about: such seemingly guiltless womanizers as Augustus John and Pablo Picasso? The public has a "sneaking regard" for their "ruthlessness" he says, but this gives evidence of being taken in by the plea of some artists for uncritical adulation by a mesmerized public. It is a strangely naive statement for an analyst who had written of defensive "self-holding" in conditions of "unthinkable anxiety". It makes one think that Winnicott conceded that full personal authenticity might not be possible, and that an omnipotent, inaccessible private self might obviate guilt and concern for others. Clearly Winnicott had not seen evidence in art of its high incidence of anxiety situations and their attempted formal, and by implication moral, resolution.

Winnicott was determined to include everything about creativity under the heading "play", even the *St. Matthew Passion.* There were to be no exclusions and, strangely, no elaboration about counteracting anxiety. Transitional objects in the potential and actual space between mother and infant were the source of all creativity: an "intermediate area which has to do with living experience and which is neither dream nor object-relating". The intermediate area is a paradox, neither object-relating nor dream: "it is neither the one nor the other of these two it is also both".[30] Lest this be thought mysticism, it should be realized that while Winnicott may have delighted in unfathomable paradox, he was no mystic seeking a unitive state. While unitive states seemed graspable to Marion Milner, and are hinted in the moments of insight she reports, Winnicott was more detached. He "knew" about, and valued, unitive mystical states but did not crave them. He wrote tentatively in 1962: "In thinking of the psychology of mysticism, it is usual to concentrate on the understanding of the mystic's withdrawal into a personal inner world of sophisticated introjects. Perhaps not enough attention has been paid to the mystic's retreat to a position in which he can communicate secretly with subjective objects and phenomena, the loss of contact with the world of shared reality being counterbalanced by a gain in terms of feeling real".[31]

This comment, made in the "counter-culture" era, was supplemented in "The Place Where We Live", with Winnicott contrasting extrovert "behaviour" with "inner" life mystical experience. "I am attempting to get in between these two extremes. If we look at our lives we shall probably find that we spend most of our time neither in behaviour nor in contemplation, but somewhere else. I ask: where? And I try to suggest an answer".[32] The answer for Winnicott himself was "in play", with words and actions having therapeutic intent, both for himself and others. Yet resolving the paradox of never being able to rest in one state or another was on his mind when he wrote of the separated baby's distress which can either be "mended" or result in traumatized "unthinkable anxiety". "This mending of the ego structure re-establishes the baby's capacity to use a symbol of union; the baby then comes once more to allow and even to benefit from separation."[33]

But what possibility is there of adult "symbols of union" dissipating the unthinkable anxiety elaborated and replicated over a lifetime? What hope is there of making such anxiety more manageable by symbolizing it in aesthetic objects? There are plenty of fear-inducing transitional gaps and voids, with imperilled objects, in Milton's epic *Paradise Lost*, for instance, and Winnicott could have studied them. It is important that Milton the poet could turn "unthinkable anxiety" over imperilled objects—Adam and Eve stalked by Satan—into life-affirming creative spaces where fallen humanity regenerates. Or, Winnicott might have thought about the many anxiety-inducing parent-child situations in Rembrandt's painting, where aesthetic containment quiets destructiveness, as in the etching of "The Return of the Prodigal Son" (1636).[34]

Winnicott seems to have been too perplexed about sex and gender to want to say much about its classical embodiments in art. Some of his least satisfactory and, one might say, anxious statements in *Playing and Reality* are about gender. Statements about split-off male and female elements seem unresolved, if not out of place, in discussions of creativity as play.[35] They amount to an investigation of, even apologia for bisexuality, which Winnicott, like Freud before him, took to be the constitutional. Winnicott speaks of "the universal acceptance of bisexuality in psychoanalytic theory" and of the fact that there is a high degree of "dissociation" in male and female identities.[36] This is taken as a given, not argued on the assumption that bisexuality might be of learned, rather than innate origin.

Winnicott knew better about himself than anyone else, and in bisexuality he may have found a limiting boundary. Bisexuality may well have been his unanalyzable "anxiety situation", not reached in Winnicott's ten-year analysis with James Strachey, or later five-year analysis with the Kleinian, Joan Riviere.[37] According to Brett Kahr, Strachey was more than a little homosexual, while his patient was "predominantly heterosexual"—a formula for unresolvable tension and anxiety between them. Breaking confidentiality, Strachey is said to have hinted to his wife, the analyst Alix Strachey, that Winnicott "suffered from erectile difficulties or even deeper terrors of the female genitalia", as Kahr puts it. Another observer suggested "total impotence", which Kahr does not find outrageous in view of Winnicott's two marriages (the first to an emotionally disturbed woman) producing no children.[38] Winnicott confessed that as a young man he had sought analysis "because I was ill".[39] After the long analysis with Strachey, the subsequent one with Joan Riviere ended unpleasantly over a difference in opinion concerning the influence of environment in child development. As late as 1962, writing to Melanie Klein, Winnicott alluded to a piece of writing he was avoiding "which touches the very root of my own personal difficulty", adding "My illness is something which I can deal with in my own way and it is not far away from being the inherent difficulty in regard to human contact with external reality".[40] Did he mean obsessive-compulsive bisexuality and, if so, was he acknowledging the end point of what he could say about creativity?

If Winnicott's was the secret of Tiresias, much is explained about his theory of creativity as "play", including the destructiveness he felt the "object" of play must survive. Resentment of dominating female influences, which might be limiting of full male sexuality, is suggested. Two sexualities, one oriented to males as passive, the other to females as active, lodged in one psyche, may be cause enough for hostility to all sexuality. Tiresias, the man-woman of legend who knew each gender's sexuality, was punished for his knowledge but ultimately became the blind seer, the wisest of men. This is paradox indeed, and it may have been Winnicott's own from which escape was impossible.

In a letter of April 15, 1966 to a female "confidant" who had just given birth, Winnicott wrote, "Everybody is bisexual in the sense of the capacity to identify with man and woman. There is a great difference, however, between a unified personality such as that of a man with a capacity for identification with a woman, and a similar but different thing, a male man with a split off woman self". He added that he was not talking about homosexuality, but "a man's woman identification".[41] He refers to gender speculations in an unpublished paper of his, which may be the grafted-on portion of "Creativity and Its Origins", in *Playing and Reality*. Here the case illustration concerns Winnicott "listening to a girl" in a male patient, and the perception having a profound effect for both analyst and patient. Winnicott's curious words are: "it is I who see the girl talking when actually there is a man on my couch. The mad person is *myself*". He continues: "This madness which was mine enabled him to see himself as a girl *from my position*. He knows himself to be a man, and never doubts that he is a man. . . . For my part, I have needed to live through a deep personal experience in order to arrive at the understanding I feel I now have reached".[42]

In writing up this case, Winnicott faced the paradox of his own Tiresias Complex, explaining the patient's sense of release following from his insights. As noted, Winnicott had been raised in a dominatingly female environment, felt guilty about a depressive mother, and attacked female dolls, which "survived". It is possible that while being outwardly accounted a boy, he had been treated somewhat as a girl, leading him to hypothesize that his patient's mother "saw a girl baby when she saw him as a baby before she came round to thinking of him as a boy". The patient "arranged his defences" according to how his mother had "failed to see him as a male".[43] As Winnicott comments, "I decided to surrender myself to whatever this might mean in myself . . . ", a confession of the first order, bearing on acceptance of bisexuality which was not homosexuality.[44] There follow speculations about the psychobiology of male and female elements in the personality, a "line of argument involv[ing] me in great difficulties . . . ", as would be expected when coming so close to his own condition.

The paper closes with perhaps Winnicott's finest piece of literary criticism in his consideration of dissociation between male and female elements in Hamlet. Hamlet tried a sado-masochistic solution to his relational dilemma with Ophelia, when in fact "there was no solution for him because of the dissociation that was taking place in him as a defence mechanism".[45] Hamlet's cruel persecution of Ophelia bespeaks his inability to accept his split off and projected female element. Knowing that it is unwise to psychoanalyze mere characters in a play, Winnicott points out that the same split gender dilemma appears in Shakespeare's sonnets, which he takes as confessional.

The conclusion of "no solution" to Hamlet's dilemma speaks for Winnicott's view of creativity in its entirety. He could have appreciated in more detail Shakespeare's, or Milton's, or Rembrandt's, insights into obsessively self-persecutory relational dilemmas and reparative impulses. He could have traced the identification of a bisexual dynamic from Tiresias to Fleiss, Freud, Havelock Ellis and others, and he could have found its painfully paradoxical working out in contemporary fiction such as that of Hermann Hesse and Ernest Hemingway. But Winnicott was not a literary or art critic. He did, however, courageously show why there could be no real and lasting "repair" of the defensively obsessive ego, turned inward toward bisexuality by stressors in primary attachment to mothers. Manic play can be more an escape that a solution, yet the "squiggle game" did tap unconscious fantasy, leading to helpful therapeutic interventions with children, and, no doubt, to relief of his own symptoms. It is regrettable that Winnicott did not pay closer attention to recurrent anxiety-laden fantasies in the productions of artists and writers. Had he done so with, say, those of the painter Francis Bacon, he could have reached insights as important with respect to homosexuality as those about Hamlet and bisexuality. But homosexuality did not that much concern

Winnicott, while bisexuality did. Winnicott's emphasis on play undoubtedly carries the risk of trivializing serious creativity and leading merely to the quixotic products of a "merry prankster", but that is to miss the true critical potential of the idea of play. Freud was right to direct attention to sexual "anxiety situations" in the psychobiographies of Leonardo and Wilhelm Jensen. Winnicott was not yet ready to follow suit, nor allow that adaptive play becomes creative (and thus reparative of, false-self solutions) only when it intersects with an anxiety situation and begins to metabolize its fear.

Notes

1. D. W. Winnicott, *Through Paediatrics to Psycho-Analysis* (London: Hogarth Press, 1975), p. 7.

   Winnicott's initial attitude to Fairbairn's revision of Freudian meta-psychology in *Psychoanalytic Studies of the Personality* was negative, as appears in a review of the book he wrote with Masud Khan. See *Psycho-Analytic Explorations*, ed. Clare Winnicott et al. (London: Karnac Books, 1989, pp. 413f. In 1967, Winnicott acknowledged his error of 1953 writing: "I now became aware that Fairbairn had made a tremendous contribution, even if we only take two things. One is object-seeking, which comes into the area of transitional phenomena and so on, and the other is this thing of feeling real instead of feeling unreal. Ibid., p. 582.

2. Winnicott, *Playing and Reality* (London: Tavistock, 1971), p. xi.

3. Brett Kahr, *D. W. Winnicott, A Biographical Portrait* (Madison, CT: International Universities Press, 1996), p. 79.

4. Ibid., p. 106.

5. Winnicott, *Playing and Reality*, p. 114.

6. Ibid., p. 114.

7. Brett Kahr, *D. W. Winnicott, A Biographical Portrait*, p.107. Winnicott was more comfortable with child fantasy than with that of adults, which included sexual anxiety.

8. Winnicott, *Playing and Reality*, p. 67, p 69. Winnicott's remarks echo Freud's famous disclaimers: "Where the artist sets his ability to create is no concern of psychology ("The Claims of Psycho-Analysis to Scientific Interest", 1913b.) and "before the problem of the poet, psychoanalysis must lay down its arms" ("Dostoievsky and Parricide", 1928).

9. Adam Phillips, *Winnicott* (London: Fontana, 1988), p. 151. See also p.145, p.149. In "Communicating and Not Communicating Leading to a Study of Certain Opposites" (1963) Winnicott had written: "In the artist of all kinds I think one can detect an inherent dilemma, which belongs to the co-existence of two trends, the urgent need to communicate and the still more urgent need not to be found. This might account for the fact that we cannot conceive of an artist's coming to the end of the task that occupies his whole nature" (*The Maturational Processes and the Facilitating Environment*. (London: Hogarth Press, 1965), p. 185).

10. Peter Fuller, *Art and Psychoanalysis* (London: Writers and Readers Publishing Cooperative, 1980), p. 164.

11. See Winnicott's "A Personal View of the Kleinian Contribution" (1962) in *The Maturational Processes and the Facilitating Environment*, p. 171f. His most telling comment is: "Klein claimed to have paid full attention to the environmental factor [in child development], but it is my opinion that she was temperamentally incapable of this" (p. 177).

12. See *The Spontaneous Gesture: Selected Letters of D. W. Winnicott*, ed, F. R. Rodman (Harvard University Press, 1987) for D.W.W. to Melanie Klein, 17 November 1952 (p. 33f); D.W.W. to Donald Meltzer, 25 October 1966 (p. 157f).

Klein tried to have it both ways writing in "On Identification": "This inner world, which can be described in terms of internal relations and happenings, is the product of the infant's own impulses, emotions and phantasies. It is of course profoundly influenced by his good and bad experiences from external sources" (*Envy and Gratitude*, p. 141). Klein had long been on record stating that "the danger arising from the inner working of the death instinct is the first cause of anxiety" ("On the Theory of Anxiety and Guilt" (1948) in *Envy and Gratitude*, p. 29). For Winnicott's struggle with Klein's concept of anxiety, depression and reparation see "The Depressive Position In Normal Emotional Development" (1954–55) in *Through Paediatrics to Psycho-Analysis*, p. 262f.

13. Winnicott, "A Personal View of the Kleinian Contribution", p. 176. See also Winnicott's comment that "I took over from [Klein], without always understanding the patterning, a very great deal which I think was original from her point of view". " But what happened to me was that I began to be interested in the environment, and this has led to something in me" ("Postscript: D.W.W. on D.W.W." in *Psycho-Analytic Explorations*, p. 576).

14. Winnicott, *Playing and Reality*, p. 70.

15. Melanie Klein, "Some Reflections on *The Oresteia*" (1963) in *Envy and Gratitude*, p. 299.

16. Winnicott, *Playing and Reality*, p. 71.

17. Clare Winnicott, "D.W.W.: A Reflection," in *Psycho-Analytic Explorations*, p. 3.

18. Ibid., p. 7.

19. Ibid., pp. 7–8.

20. Ibid., p. 8.

21. Ibid., p. 16.

22. Kahr, *D. W. Winnicott, A Biographical Portrait*, p. 10.

23. Kahr, *D. W. Winnicott, A Biographical Portrait* p. 11. See also Winnicott's "Reparation in Respect of Mother's Organized Defence against Depression" (1948) in *Through Paediatrics to Psycho-Analysis*.

24. Winnicott, "Ego Integration" (1962), in *The Maturational Processes and the Facilitating Environment*, p. 57.

25. Ibid., p. 58.

26. See *The Maturational Processes and the Facilitating Environment*, p.18, p. 41.

27. Winnicott, *Playing and Reality*, p. 41.

28. See especially "Dreaming, Fantasying and Living," *Playing and Reality*, pp. 26–7, p. 31.

29. Winnicott, "The Sense of Guilt" (1958) in *The Maturational Processes and the Facilitating Environment*, p. 26.

30. Winnicott, *Psycho-Analytic Explorations*, p. 204.

31. Winnicott, "On Communication," in *The Maturational Processes and the Facilitating Environment*, pp. 185–86. Winnicott seemed to make a concession to Milner's mystical inclination in a review of her book *On Not Being Able to Paint*: "Psycho-analysts are accustomed to thinking of the arts as wish-fulfilling escapes from the knowledge of . . . discrepancy between inner and outer, wish and reality. It may come as a bit of a shock to some of them to find a psychoanalyst drawing the conclusion, after careful study, that this wish-fulfilling illusion may be the essential basis for all true objectivity. If these moments of fusion of subject and object, inner and outer, are indeed more than islands of peace, then this fact has very great importance for education" ("Critical Notes," *British Journal of Medical Psychology*, 24 (1951): 76). Yet Winnicott's admirers do not think of him as a mystic; for instance, Peter L. Rudnytsky says simply that for Winnicott "Art provides a lifelong refuge to which we can turn as we negotiate our precarious oscillations between illusion and reality" (*Transitional Objects and Potential Spaces: Literary Uses of D. W. Winnicott* (New York: Columbia

University Press, 1993), p. xiii).

32. Winnicott, *Playing and Reality*, p. 105.

33. Ibid., p. 97. For Winnicott's view of childhood trauma see "The Concept of Trauma" in *Psycho-Analytic Explorations*, pp. 145–47. For an example of Winnicott's reparative technique in child therapy see *The Piggle: An Account of the Psychoanalytic Treatment of a Little Girl* (New York: International Universities Press, 1977). See also Rosemary Dinnage's review of *The Piggle* in which she shows Winnicott's therapy "to mend what is broken and find what is lost" (*Times Literary Supplement*, Sept. 15, 1978, p. 1025).

34. Rembrandt, *All the Etchings*, ed. Gary Schwartz (London: Oresko Books, 1977), plate B 91. In thinking about literature, Winnicott commented that fictional characters, as in novels by John Galsworthy and Leo Tolstoy, can assume blocking proportions which their authors must surmount to overcome their own anxieties (See *Psycho-Analytic Explorations*, p. 202).

35. See *Playing and Reality*, p. 72.; *Psycho-Analytic Explorations*, p. 169f for the full text of the paper read to the British Psycho-Analytical Society, 2 Feb. 1966.

36. Winnicott, "Answer to Comments" (1968-1969), *Psycho-Analytic Explorations*, p.189.

37. Kahr, *D. W. Winnicott, A Biographical Portrait*, pp. 51–52; p.61f. It is possible that Joan Riviere's thoughts about the psychological value of the performing arts may have influenced Winnicott. See her "Magical Regeneration by Dancing," *International Journal of Psycho-Analysis*, 11 (1930): 340.

38. Kahr, *D. W. Winnicott, A Biographical Portrait*, p. 45.

39. Ibid., p. 44.

40. Winnicott, To Melanie Klein, 17th November 1952, *The Spontaneous Gesture*, p. 37.

41. Winnicott, To 'M', 15th April 1966, *The Spontaneous Gesture*, p. 155.

42. Winnicott, *Playing and Reality*, pp. 73–74. See footnote p. 72 noting that the paper was read to the British Psycho-Analytic Society, 2 February 1966, and revised for publication in *Forum*. The debt to Jung's idea of pure male and female elements, animus and anima, is evident.

43. Ibid., p. 74.

44. Ibid., p. 75. Winnicott comments further, "The pure female split-off element found a primary unity with me as analyst, and this gave the man a feeling of having started to live" (p.77). Winnicott followed the psycho-analytic dogma of innate bisexuality, yet allowed that under the influence of mothering "some boys and girls are doomed to grow up with lop-sided bisexuality" (p. 83).

45. Ibid., p. 83; see also p. 84.

8

Adrian Stokes: Aesthetics, Eros and Death

Adrian Stokes (1902–1972) was the most determined and penetrating of English art critics influenced by Melanie Klein. A convinced Freudian, and later Kleinian, Stokes remained aloof from the tumultuous debates over theory that went on in his lifetime. Beginning about 1930, for seven years, he was in personal analysis with Melanie Klein, and he never departed from her basic concepts, applying them with ever increasing subtlety in his writings. So determined was Stokes to examine all the implications of Kleinianism for aesthetics and creativity, he never questioned her assumptions, for example, about paranoid-schizoid and depressive positions in infant development. This is curious as Stokes was a rigorous thinker, trained in philosophy at Oxford. He did, however, tend to take up systems as he had with F. H. Bradley's absolute idealism while an undergraduate. The question arises whether, being so uncritical of Klein and not himself an analyst lacking access to psychoanalytic debates, he forfeits credibility. In a sense, Stokes's writings on creativity are prisoners of their time, yet they also remain remarkably challenging. Winnicott, for example, considered that he had passed them by, and no doubt he did; still it is well to reconsider Stokes's contribution in some detail because it bears on the problem of anxiety as a prime motivational force in creative endeavor.[1] Further, Stokes was more than a wealthy aesthete able to please himself by living in Italy for long periods; he was a painter of some distinction.

Winnicott did not grasp that for Stokes painting was a reparative act for himself and for the acknowledged greats such as Turner and Monet—and that restoration or repair of lost or damaged objects was the painter's leading hope. So obviously right for Stokes was Klein's idea of reparation to the injured breast that he was willing to accept virtually everything else she claimed. So central was the idea of a "depressive position" (Stokes had been treated for depression) that the idea of repair simply made sense, and he readily generalized from it. As Stokes's main publicist, the philosopher Richard Wollheim, wrote: "Fear, concern, the sense of loss, a feeling for order, the desire to restore and put everything right . . . " were Stokes's leading motives.[2] The experiential source of these motives can be traced in Stokes's autobiographical "Childhood" (1947).

Both of Stokes's aesthetic and stylistic mentors, John Ruskin and Walter Pater, wrote autobiographically about their childhoods and Stokes followed their examples to good effect. He revealed for readers of his psychoanalytically informed criticism the earliest traceable states of mind necessitating concern with reparative art. The venue of an upper-middle class childhood, attended by nannies, was London's Hyde Park and Kensington Gardens. His actual household is not spoken of, and little is learned of Stokes's parents other than that his father had a serious illness when Stokes was perhaps eight.[3] The park is the focal point for all his reconstruction of feeling, not only because it contained Victorian and Edwardian statuary which he deplored. As Stokes wrote, "To explain anything we go back", and to go back to childhood in the park was for him to re-experience almost unimaginable desolation.[4]

The structure of "Childhood" is almost exactly that of the subjects in Marghanita Laski's *Ecstasy, a Study of Some Secular and Religious Experiences*: an ecstatic outcome of a series of acutely desolating childhood episodes. In her study, Laski had found, to her surprise, frequent accompaniment of ecstatic states by their opposite. Desolation-Ecstasy is not necessarily manic-depressive bipolarity in any pathological sense, but it does imply creativeness.[5] It does not seem that Stokes exaggerated the unpleasantness of his days in the London park just to emphasize what delight and deliverance had come by travelling in youth to Virgilian Italy. As he wrote of the Italian epiphany, "Existence was enlarged by the miracle of neat defining light. Here was an open and naked world. I could not then fear for the hidden, for what might be hidden inside me and those I loved. I had, in fact, incorporated this objective-seeming world and proved myself constructed by the general refulgence. Nothing, for the time, lurked, nothing bit, nothing lurched".[6] Hidden guilt and anxiety are reduced, dissipated by the Mediterranean light, and fears are repaired by pervasive aesthetic delight. But of what was Stokes afraid?

Specific experiential origins of fear and anxiety are hard to pinpoint, even in an analysis; in Stokes's Kleinian analysis they would have been assumed to be projective, not needing assignment to specific origins. This may be why Stokes does not reconstruct feelings about his parents, although he does remark on a "very strict governess", Miss Drew, who was "dismissed for maltreating me", although "I remember nothing about it". Another, Miss Harley, was "morbidly religious", and only the Swiss Mathilde was considered "fairly normal".[7] But these unpleasant relationships do not appear to be the source of his most acute suffering in the park.

Stokes was traumatized in early childhood by predatory denizens of the park he calls "parkees". It is unclear whether the assault on him was sexual, but sexual connotations surround his fears, although he is never as explicit about abuse as was Virginia Woolf in "A Sketch of the Past". Like Woolf, Stokes used both autobiographical and aesthetic means to recover lost or indistinct feelings. Of the assault Stokes writes, "Among the basins I was seized by a pack of parkees and my shouts could not be heard even a few feet away. I managed to break loose—I had the wooden handle of a push-cart with me—and regained the nurse" who had noticed nothing.[8] The parkees were probably rough boys running loose, and they left Stokes with confused, anxious and guilty feelings. "I think to this obscene hole [a tunnel in the park] I attributed the home of the animus that tore the body of the Park to shreds; the parkee spirit that made the Park poor, hungry, desolate.[9] Sexual connotations are unmistakable, as they are in a more indistinct passage about his nanny Miss Harley, who sang him guilt-inducing hymns which set off another incident that evidently left a psychological wound. Stokes writes enigmatically of "An essentially bachelor omnipresence, then, a bachelor blood-and-thunder, lay upon the slight hill beyond the Rotten Row, seared with paths like slow rolling tears of shame. He was a kind man—I understood that—this witness of all Park love-making, sexual crimes and suicides, the magician among park-keepers as he proved himself to be in the garden of Eden or in speaking from the bushes, or in hurling stone tablets out of the clouds. 'Am I my brother's keeper?' Cain had said. That was a wicked, frightened joke of Cain's".[10] Who was this false brother, and what transpired between him and the young Stokes? Stokes is not for being explicit about a probable homosexual contact, which entranced and frightened him. He speaks of "the soiled fretfulness of all happenings there each day", the park a fallen Eden in need of redemption which, in his new language, was aesthetic repair rather than Christian redemption.[11]

To Stokes, the park was "the torn, attacked and divided mother", a source of guilt and remorse needing exorcism.[12] Its description is filled with menace, dread and potential for explosive violence—exactly what would not be expected of so ruminative an aesthete as Stokes. He was deeply sensitive to the "slight, yet very frequent, traumatic experiences [which] are peculiar to the modern world".[13] From the level of his cumulative anxiety about the park it seems that Stokes's traumas may not have been so "slight". Hyper-sensitively attuned to every nuance in his environment, what to most other boys would have been passed off and forgotten was, for Stokes, residual anxiety. Realizing his vulnerability, he constructed a theory of reparative creativity to answer his need: "Each man invents a myriad states to counter his inferno. They exist abreast of the inferno; compensations, mitigations, transferences, controls, stern deletions, reparations. And so it has been with me. I have already referred to some of the priority repairs, as it were, by which the immediate patching-up was attempted. But a truly exacting person, anxious to discover a reparation of even the smallest detail, is likely to construct a state parallel to that by which inferno is summed. And indeed, it is the initial imputation, in such a strong degree, of emotional states to the external world, inferno or paradiso or both at once, that characterizes the person who will primarily be an artist, even when childhood is passed. In this, however, I do not think he is peculiar, but only extreme and exacting in the use of a compulsion commensurate with his anxiety".[14]

Stokes's hope was that "one day men will learn to think of sanity as an aesthetic achievement", but how fully was this realized?[15] A large part of his theory, especially the distinction in art between "carving" and "modelling" does not hold up to scrutiny as it assumes the correctness of Klein's unproven attribution of paranoid-schizoid and depressive features to infants. No amount of explaining "part objects" and "whole objects" makes sense of the analogy between Kleinian psychodynamics and the figurations of art.[16] As Stokes's carving and modelling theory of form and figuration in art has little explanatory power, it has not found favour in subsequent studies. Yet there is no doubt that form and imagery in painting, sculpture and architecture arise from the artist's fantasy; in anxiety Stokes had, but did not use, the key to the problem. Like Fairbairn and Winnicott, Stokes had little interest in psychobiography and so failed to follow his own best insight into the motivation behind the artistic impulse—anxiety about a threatening world.

As Stokes lacked a language of attachment, indeed of any interactive object relational theory other than Klein's, his attempts to define anxiety have a sort of philosophical complication rather than a direct bearing on experiences of himself and others with respect to art. Working with concepts and terms almost to the exclusion of affect limits his thinking to a dry theory of creativity, especially in the papers he wrote for *The International Journal of Psycho-Analysis*. Feelings of personal anxiety, so urgent in "Childhood", became a theoretical issue as he wrote for the professional journal. Only toward the end of his life did writings on aesthetics and creativity regain Stokes's rare power to convey his responses to objects that moved him and offered psychological "repair".

Stokes's struggle with negative forces of "refusal", albeit in lieu of fully espousing a "death-wish", may come as a surprise. His original idealism about art went through depressive transformations before re-emerging tempered and adjusted to the realities of mood. In "Concerning Art and Metapsychology" (1945) he spoke of art constructing "meaning", of "a synthesis of inner meaning put outwards to be on its own, as it were, in the open world . . . The artist, whatever his incapacity before the reality principle, is a self-constituted priest of Eros, the synthesizer and the object-seeker. Art is a kind of epitome, a 'useless' celebration of Eros permeating life and particularly culture".[17] Stokes may have been thinking especially of Greek culture, which ideally integrated body and mind. But, even in this paper, death obtruded: "It can . . . be argued that art is a parable of the over-all aim of human activity to force by substitutions of every kind the completeness or externality of death to serve the purposes of Eros until we die".[18] The paradox of death waiting to overwhelm life, or Eros, was to take on much larger proportions.

In "A Game That Must Be Lost" (1960), a title taken from Beaumont and Fletcher's *Philaster*, Stokes wrote that death is "the undertone of every occasion", and that the paper concerns the "threat of loss and aggression, and guilt (and eventually the later integrative processes)".[19] Stokes declares himself "on the side that favors an initial scene of inner conflict *per se*, in accordance with Freud's later theory", referring to Freud's revised theory of anxiety in "Inhibitions, Symptoms and Anxiety".[20] But had Stokes really understood the shift to object relations, to outside environmental influences, in Freud's paper? It seems not, from his insistence on an innate "danger within", menace, hate, aggression, even entropy which the instincts evolved to counteract and maintain constancy in the organism. Fear of loss, of helplessness experienced long before the emergence of sexuality and castration fears, does not impress Stokes as the prime source of depressive anxiety; so he postulates an innate "refusal", a pull toward death in every organism.

Anxiety as a correlate of a "refusal tendency", is vigorously argued in "On Resignation" (1962), resignation being advocated as a way of freeing up bound libido for "the enjoyment of the moment", even in the face of death. While there are fine words in this paper about contemplating nature as maternal and restorative, the death forces of the "refusal drive" still dominate, and we wonder how Stokes could ever return to reparative art. By 1966 the mood had softened somewhat, with Stokes writing "On Being Taken Out of Oneself". Solitude and contemplative states are advocated as producing aesthetic "refreshment" that is not outright ascetic. Stokes, however, could not decide whether "the small degree of self-annihilation at work" should be traced to "the wounds of traumatic experiences" (the emerging object relational view of Fairbairn and Winnicott) or to innate envy (Melanie Klein's view).[21] Stokes somewhat plaintively asks, "Without the hypothesis of a deadly negative principle that both persecutes and retards, and stimulates the strong yet complicated strands of the purposive in all our lives, how are we to account metapsychologically for self-persecution by guilt and remorse and for their frequent promotion of striving towards reparation, integration and truth?"[22] Unable to think outside boundaries set by Klein, Stokes had little more to offer except to say that contemplation reverses "original splitting", and offers health-giving "refusal" in place of damaging "refusal". Differing from Milner, Stokes stipulated that contemplative states were to be "an aesthetic kind in contrast with extreme or mystical forms of contemplation that aim at nothingness".[23] Antipathy to religion limited the discussion of its connection with aesthetics.

Adrian Stokes is remarkable as an art critic who freed himself from the dominant formalism of Clive Bell and Roger Fry. Bell's theory of "significant form", outlined in *Art* (1914), held that form, independent of content, was the most important feature of art, though he valued moments of aesthetic ecstasy. Stokes respected formal qualities in art, repeatedly writing about them, but he saw beyond the Bloomsbury formalist aesthetic to the energizer of art in unconscious fantasy. In Kleinianism, however, was another trap, or at least a limitation, as Stokes's thinking about creativity did not keep pace with revised developmental theory in the work of Fairbairn and Winnicott, both of whom were concerned with creativity. Just as Klein herself failed to take into account the theories of externally caused childhood trauma proposed by her teacher Sandor Ferenczi, so Stokes disregarded revisions of Freud and Klein. He did so to concentrate attention on art itself, but at a price. Further, preferring classical and Renaissance art and architecture, Stokes did not like modern expressiveness, and he especially abhorred surrealism's anarchic fantasizing. His own painting is predominantly still life and landscape, with the objects fuzzy as if just materializing—or dematerializing. It is often "inviting", but never overmastering, in its gentle, refined mystery. The bitingly expressive imagery of Alice Miller's inner world, for example, is unimaginable in Stokes's decorous aesthetic. Even the painting of his near contemporary Marion Milner is more daring in the imagery of menace it admits. For all that, Stokes's exquisite sensibility is not altogether a limitation.

Stokes's nudes are female, with the breast a prominent feature. In *Nude* (1967/8), the reclining figure's nipple is pivotal for the entire picture.[24] The nipple indeed epitomizes what Stokes called the "invitation" in art. It is hardly an unconscious manifestation, however, but charged with well-considered universal meaning. The figure's formal presentation is held in a glow of soft light that balances the maternal with the erotic. In "Reflections on the Nude"(1967) Stokes looked to the nude for "our own integration or totality, our own integration of drives and character-traits".[25] His thought was "of the mother who originally evoked our solicitude, our anxiety, as a precious whole-object that could be lost and destroyed forever".[26] Acceptance of the "good breast" was Stokes's *sine qua non* of mental health: "the good breast is the common fount of all that is good. But without a concomitant development of the good breast into the good whole-object we cannot be at home in the adult world . . . ".[27] The mother is symbolically repaired by art, reconstructed into a whole object, and other objects in the environment are ideally imbued with the feeling that they are restored good breasts—even to the point of mysticism, Stokes allowed.[28] If anything of Stokes's own history of deprivation of the breast is recorded, it has escaped search. He wrote, tellingly: "we are intact only in so far as our objects are intact. Art of whatever kind bears witness to intact objects even when the subject matter is disintegration".[29] To this he added that aesthetic experience can be defined . . . as a palliative of traumatic experience", conferring a contemplative "stillness" to allay anxieties.[30] Stokes was entirely right, but for mainly the wrong reasons insofar as he persisted with Kleinian orthodoxy.

The shift away from Klein is evident in *The Apprehension of Beauty* (1988) by the psychoanalyst Donald Meltzer, one of Stokes's closest admirers. In their dialogue "Concerning the Social Basis Of Art" (1963) Meltzer still accepted Melanie Klein's doctrine of "positions", agreeing wholeheartedly with Hanna Segal and Stokes that the artist is concerned with "the continuous process of the relationships to his inner objects, including all the vicissitudes of attack and reparation".[31] He went on to remark on Klein's discovery of projective identification of aggression and the artist's "search for freedom from anxiety and pain".[32] But influenced by the analyst W.R. Bion, Meltzer began to reconsider the origin of infant paranoid-schizoid attacks on the breast: "the thinking breast, the assimilation of the mother's eyes to her nipples, the function of her reverie in making available to the baby food for thought, the alpha-elements and dream-thoughts . . . that enable the baby to deal with emotional experiences rather than to evacuate them—none of this had worked its way into my theoretical framework or model of the mind".[33] Meltzer is hard to follow at this point in his argument, since he wanted to retain Klein's "depressive position" as "inspirational" for creative persons, at least those capable of integrating into aesthetic objects the split off elements of the ego. Melzer had noted that his most ill patients could not see beauty in objects, a function of splitting. Their persecutory anxieties as infants had less to do with innate forces, he came to think, than with whether anxiety over weaning could be successfully overcome.[34] Successfully overcome weaning anxiety traced to the quality of the mother's eyes, and how she saw her baby, Meltzer concluded. These remarks intuitively move close to attachment theory, without ever naming it.

Meltzer (and co-author Meg Williams) speculate that in idealizing the mother's body surface in nursing at the breast, infants first acquire an aesthetic sense. This is reinforced by the quality of the mother's eyes, her seeing or not seeing her baby.[35] But along with envy of her beauty, they also retain from Klein the assumption of a split off projective fear of the inside of the mother's body, which generates aggression. This situation may become dangerous for development, and holds risks of psychopathology. It also explains the life-long importance of aesthetic experience for more normal persons. It does away with Klein's assumed dramatic shift from paranoid-schizoid to depressive positions: "I think Melanie Klein was wrong to assume that a paranoid-schizoid position in object relations was anterior to the depressive position", Meltzer wrote. Instead, as Bion believed, there was a more subtle oscillation between the two emotional states, neither of which ever predominated, unless it happened that the "depressive" was actually prior to the paranoid-schizoid.[36]

By speaking of the oscillating gradations of infant-mother interactions as "aesthetic", Meltzer repositions the discussion of creativity. It is now a matter of the kind, quality and availability of the tactile and "seen" maternal breast and its substitutes. This takes us right to the verge of attachment theory's more exacting account of mother-infant interactions. Meltzer is poised to say so: "The psychopathology which we study and allege to treat has its primary basis in the flight from pain of the aesthetic conflict. The impact of separation, of deprivation—emotional and physical, of physical illness, of Oedipal conflict—pregenital and genital, of chance events, of seductions and brutality, of indulgence and over-protection, of family disintegration, of the death of parents or siblings—all these derive the core of their significance for the developmental process from their contribution as aspects of the underlying, fundamental process of avoidance of the impact of the beauty of the world, and of passionate intimacy with another human being".[37] Here, waiting to be disentangled, is virtually the whole formula for creativity in all its varieties and its anti-types. Meltzer never openly contradicted his mentor Stokes, moving beyond his into territory recognizably that of attachment theory.

Notes

1. Winnicott could be exceedingly hard on Stokes's writings on creativity, as appears in remarks to Roger Money-Kyrle, 17 March 1955:" In my view Adrian Stokes' [*Smooth and Rough*] is a sad example of an artist who struggles to cram artistic production into the introjection-projection systems and the concept of the depressive position, but the main thing that is evident is his failure since as a creative person he cannot allow it" (*The Spontaneous Gesture: Selected Letters of D.W. Winnicott*, ed. F.R. Rodman (Harvard University Press, 1987), p. 85). See also his remarks to Melanie Klein on Stokes's *Smooth and Rough* (Ibid., p. 36).

2. Richard Wollheim, Introduction to *The Image in Form: Selected Writings of Adrian Stokes*, ed. R Wollheim (Harmondsworth: Penguin, 1972), p. 10. Wollheim was a personal friend of Stokes, as he explains in "Adrian Stokes, Critic Painter, Poet," *Times Literary Supplement*, February 17, 1978, p. 207f.

3. Adrian Stokes, "Childhood," in *The Image in Form*, p.301.

4. Ibid., p. 316.

5. Marghanita Laski, *Ecstasy, a Study of Some Secular and Religious Experiences* (London: Cresset Press, 1971) pp. 166–67.

   Stokes's thoughts on creativity and trauma are found in "Some Connections and Differences between Visionary and Aesthetic Experience," in *Three Essays on the Painting of Our Time* (London: Tavistock, 1961). He writes, "All masterpieces are transfiguring if we mean by this last word that we are taken up into them. They differ in their effect from visionary objects in that they also symbolize an unchanging object- outwardness or sufficiency and an adult integration of the ego". When trauma threatens, the ego "counterattacks" which "will entail for art an increase of the symbolic use of symbolic equivalence: direct representations, either of the traumatic condition or of its cause, will yield to a symbol embracing both of them with an air of impersonality and even of 'is-ness'". (p. 43)

6. Adrian Stokes, "Childhood", p. 310.

7. Ibid., pp. 229, 301. Stokes speaks of "extreme religious fears especially for those I loved" suggesting not only fear of damnation but separation anxiety, as was typically felt by children of Stokes's class whose nurses and nannies frequently changed. (p. 301).

8. Adrian Stokes, "Childhood", pp. 291–92.

9. Ibid., p. 303. A fantasy develops of powerful sexual revulsion against nude running boys' bodies; it contains unexplained strong terms such as "suicide" and "violent dirt" (pp. 292–95). The fantasy is the opposite of a homosexually idealized painting of nude boys by Henry Tuke, for example.

10. Ibid., p. 300.

11. Ibid., p. 300.

12. Ibid., p. 294. Julia Strachey remarked with asperity on Stokes's insistence upon repairing the mother's injured breast. "He was everlastingly talking about Klein ... and how one had broken the mother. We got a bit sick really of the good breast. Either you think you've got in life a good breast or a bad breast, and if you think you got a bad breast then you sort of savage the mother ... Then afterwards you have to try and put the pieces of your mother together and that is what an artist is employed in doing ..." It was perhaps too easy to ridicule Stokes's seriousness. *Catalogue to Adrian Stokes Retrospective,* Serpentine Gallery, London, 1982 (Art Council of Great Britain, 1982) p. 21.

13. Adrian Stokes, "Cornwall and the Sense of Home," in *The Image in Form*, p. 311.

14. Adrian Stokes, "Childhood", pp. 303–4. See also the accompanying autobiographical "Living in Ticino, 1947–50", p. 317.

15. Adrian Stokes, "Living in Ticino, 1947–50," in *The Image in Form,* p. 315.

16. See for instance Stokes's "Form in Art," in *New Directions in Psycho-Analysis* (New York: Basic Books, 1955), pp. 419–20. The studies in this collection are Kleinian.

17. Adrian Stokes, "Concerning Art and Metapsychology," *International Journal of Psycho-Analysis*, 26 (1945): 177. Stokes mentions Fairbairn's theory of libido being "object seeking", but he does not develop his thoughts on this line.

18. Ibid., p. 179.

19. Adrian Stokes, "A Game That Must Be Lost," *International Journal of Psycho-Analysis*, 41 (1960):74.

20. Ibid., p. 70, p. 73.

21. Adrian Stokes, "On Being Taken Out of Oneself," *International Journal of Psycho-Analysis*, 47 (1966):524. Klein's later theory of child development added innate envy of the maternal breast to innate persecutory anxiety.

22. Ibid., p. 528.

23. Ibid., p. 529.

24. *Catalogue* to Adrian Stokes Retrospective, Serpentine Gallery, London, 1982, p. 16.

25. Adrian Stokes, *Reflections on the Nude* (London: Tavistock, 1967), p. 5.

26. Ibid., p. 5. See p. 11 for the mother's voice.

27. Ibid, p. 8.

28. Ibid, p. 12. See also "Art and the Sense of Rebirth," "The Luxury and Necessity of Painting," and "The Invitation in Art," in "The Image in Form: A Lecture"; and "Form in Art," in *New Directions in Psycho-Analysis*.

29. Ibid, p. 37.

30. Ibid., p. 50. "The Image in Form: A Lecture"

31. Donald Meltzer and Meg Harris Williams, *The Apprehension of Beauty* (The Clunie Press for The Ronald Harris Library No. 14, 1988), Addendum I, p. 209.

32. Ibid., p. 211.

33. Ibid., p. 135.

34. Ibid., p. 2; pp. 136–37.

35. Ibid., p. 60; p. 146; p. 151.

36. Ibid., pp. 26–28; See also pp. 135–36.

37. Ibid., p. 29. Earlier on this page Meltzer mentions the pioneer attachment theorist René Spitz.

9

Marion Milner: Psychoanalysis and Contemplative Creativity

Marion Milner (1900–98) is known both as an accomplished painter and as a psychoanalyst whose writings are concerned with creativity. Shaped by Freud and Klein, Milner's thinking is strongly influenced by English Romanticism, with frequent reference to such poets as Thomas Traherne and William Blake. She blends with remarkable effect continental psychological insights with an intuitive, even mystical, gift of her own. The highly individual result appeared as *On Not Being Able to Paint* (1950), a personal account of how she struggled to arrive at authentic artistic expression. Beginning with the assumption that she could paint by learning the "rules", Milner found only "a sense of emptiness and futility", as if imprisoned.[1] She had been misled by overly rational assumptions about how reality is known and had to find her way to the authentic well springs of imagination. Experiments with free association brought release but also psychological risk: "the fear that letting go common sense appearances and letting in imagination meant letting in madness".[2] *On Not Being Able to Paint* is less autobiographical than is usual in the genre to which it belongs: the English Puritan conversion narrative descending from the seventeenth century. Often using "one" when referring to herself, Milner puts distance between her actual developmental experiences and the reader. We do not hear about being parented, nor about the origins of her anxieties and fears, although as an analyzed person she had certainly confronted them. Only in *A Life of One's Own* (1934) are there glimpses of what may have been sexual abuse, from which it might be inferred that Milner's first attraction to art was escapist. But deeper knowledge of self rather than escapism became her guiding purpose. *On Not Being Able to Paint* concerns her anxiety and rebellion against authority, realized when she induced spontaneous imagery by drawing and painting. It is a conversion narrative only in the sense that it shows accessing of creative imagination by free association. Such revelation was contrary to social norms for women in 1950. Later writers on the same theme, Alice Miller for instance, would be bolder in their disclosures both of life events and in the distressed imagery in their paintings. Milner nonetheless took unprecedented risks with her own anxieties, painting and writing to discover "something of the nature of the forces that bring order out of chaos", producing integration.[3]

Milner's theorizing about creativity is incremental, growing out of enriching experiences of self through analysis and painting. Yet we are never quite certain what the "Angry Parrot"and other persecutory motifs mean in the recovered context of her life. According to Otto Rank, the artist must "play" with his or her medium to overcome a "life-fear", a prescription Milner seems to have followed. By 1956, in "Psychoanalysis and Art" she could write: "In my own attempts to study the nature of the creative process, I have become more and more aware of the anxiety which accompanies. . . deliberate reversion to a more primitive process".She realized that art had to do with contacting "forbidden wishes", and"that anxiety is not something to be retreated from, but that it is inherent in the creative process itself".[4] Freud's changing views on the sources of anxiety from inhibited sexuality to fear of separation and loss at the start of life are not mentioned, but are certainly implicit in *On Not Being Able to Paint*.[5]

Clearly Milner was interested in separation and loss, with her main concern fear of an unloved self at odds with rigid authority, possibly in excessive male will. Her book is a daring assault on the false authority of scientific reason, which may be thought of as a typically male wish to control nature. The book's most cogent feature is the suite of drawings around which she develops commentary on how producing such distressed images allowed her gradually to accept her anger against over-control. Milner describes herself as someone who naturally thinks in pictures, and an increasing facility with fantasy production is her strength. Fear of losing control is nowhere in evidence as she seems to have been able to accept and integrate even the most unexpected fantasy.

There is, however, little theory: "object relations" had not yet spoken strongly enough to Milner to risk an account of the ego organization from which she was working. Only Fairbairn's "Prolegomena to a Psychology of Art" (1938) is mentioned in the bibliography to the second edition (1957) of

On Not Being Able to Paint. In *The Hands of the Living God*, Milner notes that she waited until 1952 to read Fairbairn's paper "Schizoid Factors in the Personality" (1940).[6] This is curious as she was clearly out of sympathy with Melanie Klein's developmental assumptions leading to her theory of creativity. Milner wrote, for example, that "about 1954. . . I stopped going to Melanie Klein's seminars because I could not accept her idea of inborn envy".[7] Milner was thus cautious in using the idea of reparation, appropriate though it was to the guilt and anxiety she adduced.

She seems to have thought that Fairbairn accepted Klein's idea of "restitution" with too much alacrity, although he too doubted the underlying theory. Milner wrote cautiously of creative endeavors: "In psycho-analytic terms this process of seeking to preserve experience can certainly be described in terms of the unconscious attempt to preserve, recreate, restore the lost object; or rather, the lost relation with the object conceived in terms of the object."[8] To say "relation" was to step firmly into the object relational camp, which is where Milner belonged, especially as she came to terms with D.W. Winnicott's contributions. Discomfort with Klein (whose 1929 paper on "Infantile Anxiety Situation" is never mentioned) seems to account for Milner's backtracking when she wrote: "restoring lost objects, is in fact secondary; and that the primary role is the 'creating' of objects. . .not the recreating of them". She wrote somewhat obliquely, that the artist functions best at an earlier stage of " 'otherness' from oneself which alone makes any subsequent sadness at loss possible".[9] In other words, Milner thought that lost feelings about the past, brought on by spontaneously produced imagery, was the primary function of artistic creativity. Reparation, in the sense of restitution for guilt at primal envy of the breast, was no more in her mind than was "forgiveness" for bad mothering in Alice Miller's.

Psychoanalysts cannot be blamed for reticence but Milner's is especially conspicuous. She longed for mystical transcendence, beyond the troubles of patients, beyond the complexities of theory and beyond her own condition. There is nothing wrong with this as Milner the visualizer undoubtedly sensed primal unities behind disorganized everyday experience. Gifted with intuition which carried her beyond the sceptical reductionism too often found in psychoanalysis, Milner nonetheless resisted the lure of formal religion and of Jungianism. She sought a balance between thinking and being, between reason and emotion as appears in her best writing. Perhaps she could not have successfully treated "Susan" had she not believed that this schizoid young woman had a capacity for mystical experience: "Now at last. . . I thought I could see that Susan had been telling me something about certain aspects of the fears of mysticism as a madness. As I have said, I had found in my own experiments to do with inner awareness that the deliberate effort to wipe out all conscious imaging—verbal, visual, auditory, all images either of self or other, so that there can be a complete descent into the silent imageless existing—this was the surest way to reach an awareness of a quite different way of being from common-sense everyday functionings; and it was something that Susan had once, I felt sure, known how to do, she had spoken of it as an inner surrender to something she called God".[10]

It is clear to see why, with her intuition of primal unity beyond appearances, Milner could not remain an unquestioning Kleinian. Perhaps she was influenced by F. H. Bradley's Idealism, or she may have read Evelyn Underhill's studies of mysticism; or, maybe she was just being herself. In any case, on February 24, 1953, Melanie Klein wrote her an admonishing letter pointing out the error of thinking in terms of primal bliss. Klein wrote: "Here I come to some points where I differ from you—the feeling that these early experiences were so blissful is bound up with idealization of that baby-self and its relations, because I believe that when the baby experiences them, they are by no means free from anxieties and conflicts".[11] According to Klein, the conflict was that projective hatred was always mixed with the infant's love for its mother—an assumption Milner would not make. While not going so far as explicitly to disagree with Fairbairn's thesis that infant and child aggression is preceded by frustration in maternal caregiving, Milner's account of her patient Susan's aggression is very much in those terms. She opens the account of her case history by talking about Susan's doubts as to who her father was, difficulties with a depressed and character-disordered mother and sexual abuse by an "old man" who lived near by. With such a history there was no need to postulate primal hatred and aggression. Instead Milner began with the assumption that every person, however ill (Susan had been given ECT), has a natural integrative tendency. To evoke its healing action may take extraordinary efforts on the part of the therapist—efforts Milner was willing to make because of Susan's gift for drawing using subject matter from unconscious conflict, as she herself had learned to do. It was not that Susan projected a death wish so much as she felt she ought not to have been born at all. Yet despite Susan's bad behavior toward her therapist, Milner detected in her a wish to realign the persecutory inner world with external reality, in fact to integrate her personality.

"Restitution", or "reparation", was too limiting a term to apply to what Milner saw happening in Susan's analysis. In remarks by Lancelot Law Whyte in *Aspects of Form* (1951), Milner found better support than Klein could give for the concept of integration, and of bridging inner with outer reality. As Milner explains, "During this time [of Susan's analysis] I was also preoccupied with what I then called the spontaneous urge to pattern inherent in the living organism; also with the possibility that a number of states of mind that are different from everyday conscious awareness may be related to the need to give this inner organizing force full play; in addition there was the idea that this form of organization comes about not by planned action, but only by a planned framework, within which the free play of unplanned expressive movement can come about, what I came to call 'contemplative action'.[12] Milner thus brilliantly joins the biological concept of persons as self-organizing naturally integrating systems, with "play" which frees up the process of integration, along with reflection or contemplation, by which play actions are transformed into lastingly available enriched feelings of relatedness. This formulation could not be more important, and while not explicitly addressing the question of anxiety being the motivating factor requiring integration, it does typify the argument of this study of creativity in its entirety. By providing a "holding environment", Milner allowed Susan play in drawings and verbalizings which reduced anxious aggression, thereby improving integration and lessening her schizoid condition. *The Hands of the Living God* is as strong a testimony to the healing powers of creativity as has been recorded.

Milner's idea of "contemplative action", allied to mysticism in creativity, also helps to explain her differences with D. W. Winnicott, with whose thinking she mainly agreed. In "Playing: Creative Activity and the Search for the Self", however, Winnicott arrived at a conclusion which Milner could not accept. According to Winnicott, "In a search for the self the person concerned may have produced something valuable in terms of art, but the successful artist may be universally acclaimed and yet have failed to find the self that he or she is looking for. . . . If the artist . . . is searching for the self, then it can be said that in all possibility there is already some failure for that artist in the field of general creative living. The finished creation never heals the underlying lack of sense of self'.[13] By contrast, Milner thought that an improved "sense of self" could be achieved by "play" with the elements of reverie and imagination, and that it could be "contacted" in conscious life. She wrote: "Certainly I had found that there is a contact that can result in a renewal, a rebirth; provided, that is, that one is prepared to stop the inner chatter of introspective arguments and face the inner silence, the basic formlessness from which all form comes, and which at first can feel like total emptiness, annihilation even, and be defended against at almost any cost".[14] Milner did not mean "the phantasy of the destruction of the inner needed object", but the coinciding of two circles (a motif in her own painting and in Susan's drawing) "till they coincide as a single circle; in fact, a unity which can be seen as either everything or nothing, as a total eclipse of the sun, a dark night of the soul, or a blissful consummation".[15] In other words, to find a self, one must first surrender to silence and otherness, cease pressured seeking and "let be". Such mystical awareness is not to be found in the busy verbalizations of Winnicott's insistence on maintaining "paradox", a tension of opposites that could never be reconciled. No other analyst was willing to go as far as Milner in crediting mystical awareness with healing powers. Mysticism in world religions was discredited mainly by analysts in the Freudian tradition, who sceptically assumed origins in inhibited sexuality. Milner did not engage in argument with the sceptics, choosing to go her own way as artist-analyst.

Suffice it to say that Milner and Winnicott were so temperamentally different that their presuppositions do not really coincide, Milner believing in a primal unity inaccessible to Winnicott. "Play" and "sense of self" had different meanings, although it is clear that Milner made no claim that artistic creation itself constituted any sort of final achieved unity of the personality. If such was to be, it lay beyond the artistic endeavor, a preparatory set of exercises at best. As she wrote in a note, a seeming afterthought but central to this discussion, Milner agreed with Adrian Stokes, and with Anton Ehrenzweig who spoke of art as the receiving womb, a place of integration and rebirth, that art is not the final achievement. "The finished work was more . . . an encouragement to the ego; that is, as I saw it, an enshrining of an ideal integration, rather than necessarily a permanent internal achievement of it".[16] This sounds more like Winnicott's limiting statement about creativity, but it is quite compatible with Milner's acceptance that to create and to heal, one must stop trying and let unnamed, inherent organizing forces take over.

In her own right, Milner was a discoverer of the unconscious, probing her experience in two pre-World War II books: *A Life of One's Own* (1934) and *An Experiment in Leisure* (1937). So daring for a woman were these writings that Milner chose to use a pseudonym, Joanna Field. She wrote to overcome the restrictions of a Church of England belief system and to surmount the growing dominance of scientific rationalism among intellectuals; but most of all she wrote to free herself from fear of non-being. She began keeping a diary at age twenty-six and continued about seven years when her first book took shape. The diary form, which descends in England through Puritan spiritual account keeping, is an immediate means of recording episodic events, along with feelings and reflections upon them. Diaries tend to be directionless, disconnected and shapeless. Milner pulled together her material with as much meaning as she could give it and, if present-day readers have questions she hadn't considered, or suspect conclusions she couldn't draw, she is hardly to be faulted given her achievement in "experimenting" with authenticity of feeling at the time.

Bound by a "tradition of reticence", Milner "shrank from the thought of a direct personal account of what happened to me, yet knew all the time that only as such could it have any value to others".[17] *A Life of One's Own* is certainly disappointing in that little is said of Milner's parenting and development; while knowing that confession of shameful feelings is "cleansing", "I knew then that though my decision to write in direct personal terms would lead me on to dangerous ground yet it was the very core of my enterprise".[18] She could of course have conveyed her personal story as fiction, but by neither fictionalizing nor writing straight autobiography, which might have been hurtful to living persons, Milner was restricted to a sort of inner-life review that can be opaque. That is not to deny that it frequently comes startlingly alive, only that the full life context is missing so that readers cannot judge the appropriateness of strong emotions discovered beneath the decorousness of an early twentieth century young English woman of the educated upper middle class. In this respect Adrian Stokes's revelation of childhood fear and desolation is much to be preferred, yet Stokes lacks Milner's genius for lucid, detailed introspection, being quicker to take refuge in the Kleinian theory which she would eventually reject.

Despite lack of circumstantial detail, suggestions of unmastered trauma —in imagery of ghouls and dragons—are present in Milner's diary, giving the background of anxiety from which an interest in creativity might grow: "So one day when I was feeling particularly under a cloud of apparently causeless anxiety I wrote: 'Why this uneasiness? foreboding?—doing wrong —punishment—that I'll be found out—I call it selfishness—I feel I'm missing something and always feel it's not for me to do the things for other people, but when I do then very often I'm happy. . .a woman's breasts—a bird's nest, all soft and smooth feathers—the little white underneath parts of a dormouse. What's this got to do with now?' and so on, ending up with: 'a black man holding you, a baby, in his arms, up in a tree—black man—father—he must have nursed me as a baby—I remember his study with the sparking coil and his singing me to sleep—'Now the day is over'". The passage is deeply enigmatic, with no explanation of a "black" father (although it should be remarked that her maiden name was Blackett), of absence of mother, or of the association with female adult sensuality. Milner's puzzled comment is: "Although I could not then tell what all this meant, it was clear that my automatic [unconscious] self was busy with happenings in my remote past and was perhaps bringing over into my present concerns emotions which had no real connection with adult life. Certainly I had not seen the electrical machine in my father's study since before I was three years old. What connection this had with my present anxieties I could not see".[19] While Milner goes on to speak of dreaming of the sea as mother, her free associations quickly deflect to God, bringing a flood of malign, persecutory associations to the idea of fatherhood. Free association lifts raw, unprocessed material from the unconscious, but she cannot do more than record an amorphous mass of fantasy in which God is both persecutor and saving parent.

A few selected passages convey contradictory, dire and unmetabolized feelings: "Oh God, help us—be merciful unto us, miserable sinners—shall we never escape from the body of this death—grow old along with me, the best—they said you'd be raped by tramps on the grassy hills—I cried—Oh God, is it come to this—Lord save us—what from?"Later the associations run, "crawling worms and mud—blind sea worms . . . hateful—menstruation —the hellish smell of blood—the end of everything—Prison—prison—skirts hampering—hairpins—hateful—humorous—laughter jokes—nasty—dirty —foul smells—sweaty bodies—a man's healthful body— shirt open—P— vigour and happiness—freedom—damn the God of your Fathers—blasphemy —my God is better than. . . . " Still later the picture darkens again as Satan replaces God: "Devil—D—Dad—down—duty—downpour—this is rot—rot —rotting—decay—death—. . .a personal villain . . . —Pleasure—Lust—decay —whoreson—disease—plague—putrefaction" etc. Mention of "gin—grog. . .and blue frocks and tense voices", suggests drinking and sex. And most disturbingly, Milner pictures God as having power to put one "in a cage and you can't escape"; "God said this must be—so said one's parents—why, why, why, why—I hate God—God doesn't want me to be happy—'Why must I do it?'—'Because I say so'—and who are you?—why I should I obey you? —I won't, I won't, I won't—child . . . it's doing it because you love it — love, love, like the moments of joy in people and beauty and shape . . . love is of God".[20] Who can say that the child Marion Blackett was sexually abused, let alone by her father—because, as far as I know, she has never expressly said so? The powerful fantasy language of these passages, leading to the conclusion that Milner's anxiety had specific traumatic causes of which she could tolerate only partial awareness, makes this a viable hypothesis.

The existence in her diary of tormented and dissociated passages on God, Satan and implied sexual violation helps to explain why Milner did not cast *A Life of One's Own* as conventional narrative. She could not give narrative form to recovered traumatic experience which remained emotionally unmetabolized. That the dissociated passages were not altered or removed attests to their centrality, but neither do they seem more fully understood in "twenty-five years of living", and in the sixteen years between publication and re-issue of the book. On the latter occasion Milner wrote, "During this time the main issues have gradually become clearer; I have, however, made no substantial alteration in this book".[21] Nor does her 1986 discussion of reviews of the book show that the passage on sexual abuse had been picked up, nor that sexuality (other than the theme of bisexuality) had impressed readers. Sexual abuse had not yet been enough revived as an issue in psychodynamic theory, nor does Milner seem to have worked with Freud's early ideas about the traumatic origins of hysteria. Milner did not enter the controversy over real and imagined paternal abuse of daughters.

Contrasting passages of the most captivating visionary experience also occur in the narrative, giving it literary distinction. Smooth, gathered and coherent in contrast to the rough, broken and dissociated diary material on abuse, the visionary passages are too frequent to be chance events. They are the saving staple of Milner's inner life, cultivated and directed by the discipline she learned. They are regenerative, reparative emotional "inscapes" (as the poet Gerard Manley Hopkins termed union between the poet's heightened awareness and the "isness" of natural objects). An example is Milner's seeing swans on a pond in Golders Hill Park in London, an experience which acquired "a 'thusness', 'so and no other wise' existing in an entirely different sphere from the world of opinion".[22] Her discovery of "a more vivid power of perceiving came in the Black Forest, Germany where "a simple incantation" about seeing ordinary objects "seemed to open a door between me and the world" such that "I sat motionless, draining sensation to its depths, wave after, wave of delight flowing through every cell in my body".[23] Such experiences are perhaps unsurprising revivals of English Romantic consciousness from William Wordsworth's narrative poem "The Prelude" (1805) to Richard Jefferies's autobiographical *The Story of My Heart* (1907), both pantheistic, as Hopkins's poetry tended to be. Unlike the visionary landscapes of William Blake and Samuel Palmer, Milner's verbalized visions are without human figures, completely "safe spaces" where anguish and guilt cannot enter. They are clarifying "openings", not the confusing "closures" of the diary fantasy of God, the dangerous but saving father.

Milner well knew that psychoanalysts were apt to question the validity of mystical experiences as simply hysterical evasions of reality. In *An Experiment in Leisure* (1937), she remarks that Herbert Silberer's *Problems of Mysticism and Its Symbolism* had reminded her that mental images might be merely "'wish-fulfilments', as a means of evading hard facts; but [the mind] also uses them as a way of thinking about hard facts; as an instrument, not for the evading of truth, but for reaching it".[24] There is no doubt that Milner's anxiety, guilt and depression were modified by visionary experiences toward healthy re-engagement with life. Her moments of heightened awareness were not simply evasions, or escapist compensations for suffering with which she could not constructively work. (It would be important to know what her Freudian analysis with Sylvia Payne produced along these lines, but Milner's writings are silent on that matter.) The point about her writings is that they discover a reliable method of mood control, of neutralizing anxiety and depressive affect—reversing the sense of non-being that was due to more than the subordinate place of women in Milner's England. A claim could be made for Milner's "doodling" and "free writing", done without conscious control that, not only did they open channels of communication within herself, they also discovered the 'relaxation response', explained recently in medical terms by Herbert Benson. Her method of "letting go" so that imagery arises is very close to Buddhist Vepassena meditation, and her "watching" of the inner life resembles the attachment theorist Mary Main's idea of "metacognitive monitoring" which also enlarges the inner life.[25]

It may be doubted that Milner ever connected, through the example of Jungian archetypes or any other psychodynamic means, the terrors of sexuality with the healing sublimity of dreams and visions of nature. The two seem to stand in contrast in her writings, their connection left in question for the reading public. *An Experiment in Leisure* clarifies her "ritual sacrifice" method of relaxing will, striving for results invariably producing "the clutch of anxiety", and feelings of inferiority.[26] She addresses the problem of female masochism, and indeed the book seems more-feminist than her later psychoanalytic writings. There is useful discussion of depression, the ambiguity of gender and of the power of older women to intimidate younger ones.[27] There is an eloquent plea for letting the unconscious do its imaginative work by "the plunge into the abyss", but there are no imaginative enactments to show early traumatic experiences being integrated into the perplexities of adult relationships.

For Milner, herself an artist, the finished work of art being able to heal an underlying lack of sense of self was not an issue. She knew that art alone could not heal, but it could release healing forces that operate beyond art. Twentieth century scepticism about the language of self-transcendence into 'nothingness' where healing energies generate, kept her reticent in later years. But clearly Milner continued learning about self-transcendence from such mentors as the poet and painter William Blake and from Zen masters. Her ultimate category of meaning in transformed moments of awareness is clear throughout her writings on creativity, and it is made experiential in her personal diaries and reflections. She writes in *Eternity's Sunrise*, for example: "If atheists are people who say there is nothing there, only emptiness, could it be that they have got hold of half of a truth, only misinterpreted it, refused to relate themselves to that nothingness?"[28]

Her responses to nature and art are of awed silence at the wonder of creation. She finds revelation without the trappings of any system of religious belief. But there are certain limitations too: Milner might have examined in more detail the psychoanalytic objection that mysticism traces to inhibited sexuality being avoided by idealization of a distant but possibly nonexistent 'good object'. She would rather dwell on contemplative states—moments of being—induced by nature and art than theorize about the difficulties we know she had. In writing of moments of heightened being, Milner's work gives a sense of incompleteness. Where in her art and writing are the desolation experiences that must have accompanied the ecstacies? A reviewer of her early books noted of Milner that "she had periods of acute anxiety, a feeling of being cut off from other people, and—most disturbing of all—a growing sense that her life was not her own".[29] The theme of overcoming personal anxiety is not carried over into Milner's mature writings on creativity. This contrasts sharply with Virginia Woolf writing "A Sketch of the Past" of how "separate moments of being were however embedded in many more moments of non-being".[30] Woolf is more circumstantial than Milner in her search for "wholeness"and "pattern" behind the flux of experience. Loss of her mother by death is brilliantly evoked in images of empty black spaces, a sort of atmospheric recreation of the Stephen household, and of personal non-being. For Woolf, "Many bright colours; many distant sounds; some human beings, caricatures; comic; several violent moments of being, always including a circle of the scene which they cut out: and all surrounded by a vast space—that is a rough visual description of childhood".[31] Woolf fell too soon into suicidal depressive desolation, while Milner triumphed over desolation to enter a remarkably serene old age. But the exact biographical conditions of Milner's creativity remain obscure, unless she too leaves a "Sketch of the Past", concerning "whatever problems had worried me even from the very earliest years of childhood".[32]

Notes

1. Marion Milner, *On Not Being Able to Paint* (1950) (London: Heinemann, 1971), p. 91. Psychoanalysts generally welcomed this highly original book. Ronald Fairbairn welcomed it for discussing creativity "wholly in terms of object relationships", while Donald Winnicott commended it for recognizing the illusions of art, which are really a source of objectivity, and for commending "the role of spontaneity in creativeness". Only Michael Fordham took exception: "one would have

expected a more radical attempt to analyse the original conflict in relation to infancy". Fordham's remark is accurate as Milner did not offer a full self-disclosure of the creative urge traced to earliest infancy and childhood (*British Journal of Medical Psychology*, 24 (1951): 72; 76; 75).

2. Ibid., p. 17.

3. Ibid., p. 148.

4. Marion Milner, *The Suppressed Madness of Sane Men: Forty-four Years of Exploring Psychoanalysis* (London: Tavistock, 1987), pp. 211–12. Rank's remarks on "life fear" are found, for example, in *Art and Artist*, p. 101.

5. Marion Milner, *On Not Being Able to Paint*, p. 57.Separation and loss are central concerns, and Milner reflects how the painter can externalize in imagery what was anxiously taken inside the psyche to forestall loss. She also reflects on the danger of enveloping anxiously internalized objects (p. 63).

6. Marion Milner, *The Hands of the Living God: An Account of a Psycho-Analytic Treatment* (New York: International Universities Press, 1969) n.2, p. 245.

7. Marion Milner, *The Suppressed Madness of Sane Men*, p. 292. See also *The Hands of the Living God*, p. 255.

8. Marion Milner, *On Not Being Able to Paint*, p. 159.

9. Ibid., p. 160.

10. Marion Milner, *The Hands of the Living God*, p. 408. "We had even seen the struggle leading to [Susan's] battles over the nature of creative thinking, up to her slow recognition of that opposite of her conscious thinking that is unconsciousness, the gap in unconsciousness that consciousness has to relate itself to, the something not there, the Cloud of Unknowing, the empty Circle" (p. 461–62). Milner not only felt that Susan's schizoid split between aggression and tenderness was healing,

and that concern for Milner as a real person was emerging, but that a healthy capacity for self-transcendence was also developing, and not as mere escape. (pp. 398–99).For the "blankness or gap in one's perception" helpful in creativity see *The Suppressed Madness of Sane Men*, p. 260. Milner pays tribute to Anton Ehrenzweig's idea that mysticism comes of the disjunction between surface and depth perception, and reports finding "in my own experiments, that the deliberate effort, at times, to wipe out all conscious imaging—verbal, visual, auditory—and to descend into awareness of an imageless existing, within one's own body, this could result in a way of being that was not only highly recuperative but also a great enrichment of one's appreciation of the outer world" (p. 263). That Milner was aware of Zen Buddhism appears in *The Hands of the Living God*, p. xxvi.

11. Marion Milner, *The Suppressed Madness of Sane Men*, p. 109.

12. Marion Milner, *The Hands of the Living God*, p. 263. Milner's appendix of terminology used in Susan's case includes "Reparation"as defined by Hanna Segal (a follower of Melanie Klein), p. 419, and "Integration"as defined by Melanie Klein, p. 419. From the early 1950s Lancelot Law Whyte published various speculations about the biology of form, culminating in *Accent on Form: An Anticipation of the Science of Tomorrow* (1973). Grounded in science as Klein's were not, Whyte's views compelled Milner to rethink the idea of form as inherent in all life.

13. D.W. Winnicott, *Playing and Reality* (London: Tavistock, 1971), pp. 54–5.

14. Marion Milner, *The Suppressed Madness of Sane Men*, p. 109.

15. Ibid., p. 284.

16. Marion Milner, *The Hands of the Living God*, p. 410, note 1.

17. Joanna Field [Marion Milner], *A Life of One's Own* (London: Virago Press, 1986), p. 32.

18. Ibid., p. 32.

19. Ibid., p. 61.

20. Ibid., pp. 62–4. See also p. 66 for how free association revealed ambivalence about an attractive man.

21. Ibid., Prefatory note to the 1952 edition.

22. Ibid., p. 49. See also, for example, "half-opened leaves", p. 49; the Cézanne still life, p. 76; seeing Cornwall afresh, p. 77; the Mediterranean sea scape and the cyclamens, p. 107, with visionary experience discussed pp. 103f, p. 198.

23. Ibid., pp. 78–9.

24. Joanna Field [Marion Milner], *An Experiment in Leisure* (Los Angeles: Jeremy Tarcher, 1987), p. 50.

25. See *A Life of One's Own* for "free writing", p. 166, p. 181, pp. 190–1; for dreams and dreaming, p. 150, p. 162; relaxation response, p. 175, pp. 192–3; mindfulness, pp. 179–80; communication as health-giving, pp. 194–5.

26. Marion Milner, *An Experiment in Leisure*, p. 40.

27. Ibid., pp. 197–8.

28. Marion Milner, *Eternity's Sunrise: A Way of Keeping a Diary* (London: Virago, 1987), p. 119.

29. Linda Gerend, "Moments of Delight," *Times Literary Supplement*, December 19, 1986, p.119.

30. Virginia Woolf, "A Sketch of the Past," in *Moments of Being*, ed. J. Schulkind (New York: Harcourt Brace, 1976), p.70.

31. Ibid., p. 79.

32. Marion Milner, *A Life of One's Own*, p. 147.

10

Alice Miller: Creativity as Insight

"Probably everybody has a more or less concealed inner chamber that he hides from himself and in which the props of his childhood drama are to be found", wrote Alice Miller, whose studies of creativity center on overcoming childhood traumas.[1] An ex-Freudian analyst, Miller sets out her theory of emotional suffering as originating in actual mother-child interactions. Having forsaken drive theory, and avoided the dogmas of Melanie Klein, Miller would seem to have entered the arena of real-life experience occupied by attachment theorists. Yet she appears to be an independent discoverer rather than a follower of John Bowlby. She draws on her own experience of childhood suffering and on the disappointment of fruitless Freudian search for relief from oppressive mothering. Strongly autobiographical, Miller has yet to publish a full account of childhood deposits in her own "inner chamber". Her argument for relief from suffering through creativity draws on spontaneous imagery without the encompassing "story", but it is nonetheless powerful.

Reacting against dogmatic Oedipal theory, Miller shows by the evidence of her own distraught imagery in paintings how the residues of over-controlling, "pedagogic" mothering cause suffering that escapes the analytic method. Free association, Miller asserts, cannot reach the level of psychological organization where manipulative mothering registers but results instead in overly intellectualized verbal interaction with the analyst. *Pictures of a Childhood* (1986) presents in sixty-six watercolors the evidence for having contacted the damaged inner child that two formal Freudian analyses had failed to contact. It is, of course, possible that poetic creativity might have revealed the same suffering, vindicating free association, but Miller chose non-verbal imagery, reminiscent of Marion Milner's, to probe the inner chamber of conflicted childhood feelings. Her method answers to Henri Ellenberger's idea of inducing a "creative illness" more than it does to any established therapeutic method, and it is doubtful that Miller could have fully contacted childhood feelings without the discipline of the analytic training she so denigrated. Nevertheless, the stunning result has the power and originality of products of Freud's and Jung's own creative illnesses as described by Ellenberger.[2] The profusion of imagery Carl Jung produced in his "confrontation with the unconscious" in the crisis period of 1913 was not "art", he decided, but spontaneously arising archetypes of the unconscious. The visionary rebirth he underwent, with all the pyrotechnics of a cosmic upheaval, he calls a "solar myth" of the hero, linked to a review of life events to be sure, but nonetheless displaced onto the cosmos.[3] Miller had no such cosmic consciousness, mentions no archetypes and avoids the philosophical problem of "innate ideas" posed by Jung's theory. Yet Miller and Jung share a concern with the emotionally perilous mother, for Jung the cunning anima "mouthpiece of the unconscious", who "can utterly destroy a man", and for Miller her own mother, "a brilliant pedagogue, [who] succeeded perfectly in crushing my true feelings and needs in such an imperceptible way that neither I nor anyone else realized what had happened".[4] Miller's watercolors are not "art" either, except in the broadest sense of products of creativity: they are pictographs of isolation, menace and suffering, of chronic inner distress and rage at imprisoned feelings. They release the feelings from their impounded state by vibrant colors and emphatic black lines delineating tense and destructive forces. There is no narrative context, titles are not supplied nor is the exact sequence established by dates. The viewer is confronted by the pictures to guess at actual childhood events and the residues of feeling states needing integration into conscious awareness.

Miller's method may have been suggested by Winnicott's "squiggle game", often used with brilliant effectiveness in child analyses—spontaneous cooperative drawing between child and therapist—but much more Miller drew upon the discoveries of early modern painters such as Picasso, Miro, Paul Klee and Chagall.[5] Of historical painters she praises Turner, Goya and Cézanne "for going ways that were unfamiliar to others but essential for themselves".[6] Derivative though her techniques and even imagery may be, the paintings authentically come across as revived from sources as early as childhood. They have the energy and flow of spontaneous creations by someone steeped in modern art yet deeply in touch with lost feelings. They are indeed images of anxious attachment generalized to a communicable level but retaining the rudiments of an actual story of childhood development. The viewer "knows what they mean" without the detailed self-diagnosing that might arise should Miller publish her autobiography in an undisguised form.

There is no disputing the validity of archetypes which, sooner or later, come into play in artistic creativity. They may be ignored or emphasized, but when they arise from the unconscious, they give art special resonance. Jung perhaps took refuge in archetypes from the too painful actualities of attachments to father and especially to mother, while Miller minimized them to emphasize childhood suffering alone. It was no doubt inevitable that such a shift from spirituality to hard realism would occur as it had been in process through the entire modern period in Europe. The search for authentic encounter with childhood experience is very evident throughout the arts of this period. Yet the advance is often hesitant and guarded, with indirection the rule in the arts. For example, the Bauhaus teacher and painter Wassily Kandinsky's *On the Spiritual in Art* clearly wanted to talk about childhood: "Every work of art is the child of its time; often it is the mother of our emotions". Kandinsky goes on to condemn materialism, predict "emerging soul" and call on the artist to "give free scope to his feelings . . . the spiritual necessity of nascent awakening."[7] His extraordinarily dynamic early compositions are evidence that Kandinsky had tapped into unconscious energies previously held under greater control by artists. Paul Klee, Kandinsky's Bauhaus colleague, not only stated that he painted from the unconscious, but he kept a diary of inner experience from 1898, when he was 19. The diary opens with thirty-seven paragraphs of "Memories of Childhood"; from age two onward apprehensions of death, evil-spirits and early sexual anxieties are prominent. In his Jena lecture of 1924, Klee wrote "Our heart . . . urges us to go deeper, down to bedrock. What comes of this impulse—however you call it: dream, idea, imagination—is not to be taken seriously until it has been given bodily shape in the work of art, through the creative procedure that is suited to it".[8] This is exactly Miller's program in her painting, as spontaneous image-making is shown to give more certain access to primal emotional states than words can do. There was plenty of inducement in the culture to formulate childhood experience such as Franz Kafka's "Letter to His Father" (1919) and Hermann Hesse's "Childhood of the Artist"(1923) but the painters worked still closer to unacknowledged feelings, refraining from formulating them in words while letting them emerge through freely invented imagery and profusions of color. Miller tells us that

"Five years after I began to paint, I started writing my books which would never have been possible without the inner liberation painting had given me".[9] In other words, all Miller's teachings about psychopathology having its source in emotional abuse in childhood arose from her discovery of having been an abused child herself—unknown until forcefully given back by her own creative imagery. Spontaneous imagery unerringly found the locus of primal anxiety in the mother-daughter relationship, delivering it for re-processing in a new self-aware mode. Miller says explicitly that creativity gives "form to the chaos within us and thereby allows us to master our anxiety".[10] Mastering our anxiety is exactly the insight Freud brought out in "Inhibitions, Symptoms and Anxiety" (1926), his response to Otto Rank's theory of the birth trauma. Contrary to Rank, Freud showed that anxiety can arise through any apprehension of loss of mother or distortion of caregiving in the developmental process. The child's traumatized ego actively repeats the trauma but in a weakened version in the hope of overcoming its unpleasantness. Anxiety is counteracted by reparation which is activated in patients who go on to therapeutic success. Miller seems to have forgotten Freud's insights into the core developmental problem which she evoked in her paintings of small and vulnerable beings in threatening fields of force, for example, illustrations 10, 14, 21, 25, 34, 44 and even the comparatively reconciled 66, in which the child's mouth is covered and the frightened eyes register anxiety over merger with the mother. Miller writes persuasively about narcissistic conditions arising from failures of mothering when the child lacks "a reliable framework for emotional checking to his symbiotic partner".[11] This is the language of attachment taking its inspiration from Freud's insights of 1926 and anticipating Bowlby's expansion to the point of supplanting psychoanalysis itself.

Miller's campaign against orthodox psychoanalysis throughout her writings has an unfortunate effect on the entire enterprise. While undeniably Freud's 1897 abandonment of the trauma theory of hysteria called for reconsideration, Miller's attack seems virulent. Only Geoffrey Masson's disillusioned discovery that Freud continued "seeing the reality of sexual abuse in his own private practice, after he had supposedly abandoned the theory" attains the intensity of Miller's denunciation.[12] That Freud should self-protectively allege that hysterical women had made up stories of sexual abuse needs balanced assessment in the light of more recent trauma studies. But for Miller it led to a campaign against psychoanalysis only softened by occasional glances at

Freud's own childhood suffering. From her opening note to *The Drama of the Gifted Child* (1979)—"I have become more and more suspicious of the validity of Freudian drive theory and have re-experienced a growing need to distinguish between it and my own views"[13] to *Banished Knowledge: Facing Childhood Injuries* (1990), she wages a campaign against drive theory as an instrument of "poisonous pedagogy". Psychoanalysis is a "maze of well-tended paths but with no exit into freedom", a useless intellectualizing of suffering that has quite other causes than those Freud alleged in Oedipal theory, she writes.[14] Certainly this needed saying as it does of any overly rigid system using dogma to resist revision.

But for all its limitations psychoanalysis had been a liberating force to which Miller owed the beginning of her own emancipation. Her excessive attack on Freud's theory as a defensive system in itself, seems to be an attack on the father whose absence from Alice Miller's account of her own quest is its most puzzling feature. Even if he only planted a seed and was thereafter completely absent, the father must be accounted for. Father absence often leads to childhood fantasies of hero or villain fathers, or some mix of the two, which need to be explicit in a full account of creativity. At least we need to know what feelings about men the unconscious discloses by its unerring imagistic messages. Miller had hoped by her art to "let the child lead me", to "speak the language of the unconscious" and thereby revive a threatened "authentic self".[15] Clues to Miller's childhood traumas appear in the semi-autobiographical *Paths of Life: Seven Scenarios* but they are not connected to the question of artistic creativity. How can Miller's theory of creativity be accepted as the true new direction, acknowledging the causality of childhood trauma, when the full data of her creative illness are not offered and the contributing theories are inadequately considered?

Miller is hard on analysts who would seem to be her allies, Sandor Ferenczi, for example. For his enunciation of the primacy of trauma-causing child abuse Ferenczi was ejected from Freud's inner circle. One would think that such a martyr to now substantiated truths would be celebrated by Miller, but that is not what we find. Ferenczi may have tried to free himself, but both he and Robert Fliess "remained locked in the prison of psychoanalytic concepts", she writes—an instance of metaphor standing in for scholarship as Miller seems not to have read Ferenczi's last and most brilliant paper on child abuse, "Confusion of Tongues . . . " (1932), nor his confessional *Clinical*

Diary [16]. Her negative view if Melanie Klein's "theory of the cruel infant", and of Freud's drive theory, which was aligned with the "traditional pedagogic view of the child", is more considered and just.[17] Miller is among the first major theorists to reject out of hand Klein's primacy in this area of psychoanalytic thought. In rejecting her, however, Miller also neglects the critical question of what constitutes "anxiety situations" which had she considered them as such would have led her back to Freud. Instead she leaps forward to a new set of theorists—initially to D.W. Winnicott, Margaret Mahler and Heinz Kohut, then to Arthur Janov and later to René Spitz, John Bowlby, Lloyd deMause and Frederick Leboyer.[18] Differing widely in profession, attitude and emphasis with respect to psychoanalysis, these theorists share a concern with the effects and meaning of childhood trauma. Only Bowlby, assisted by the Robertsons' early observational studies of infant and child separation, advanced the science of attachment to a level confirming Miller's assertions. Her theory of creativity as inducing mourning for failures of infant and childhood attachment, which necessitates recovery of repressed feelings of actual early experience, exactly complements Bowlby and his followers' work on attachment.[19] Miller speaks of "recovered long repressed anxiety" as a prelude to healing mourning —virtually formulating, independently it seems, John Bowlby and Mary Ainsworth's theory of "anxious attachment" arising from circumstantial failures in the mother-infant nexus. Miller was on the track of genuine advance in the theory of creativity but without joining forces with those she saw as her closest allies. Instead, Miller recommended the self-directed therapy of J. Konrad Stettbacher, whose four-step procedure is given in *Making Sense of Suffering: The Healing Confrontation with Your Own Past* (1991). This self-help book does not try to advance theory of creativity but to directly help persons to discover and reconstruct childhood events implicated in adult suffering.

Miller's lack of engagement with attachment theory may account for the comparative paucity of her efforts in extended psychobiography of creative persons and the disappointing results of her applied studies. With the enormous advances in understanding infant and child development, particularly following from John Bowlby's *Attachment and Loss* (1969f), it is to be wondered that Miller's study of childhood suffering in creative persons does not make explicit use of them. The fullest and most astute of Miller's psychobiographies is of Franz Kafka in *Thou Shalt Not Be Aware: Society's Betrayal of the Child*

(1986). It observes that Kafka was dreaming as he wrote out "his anger at not being understood", and the victim of repressed feelings that depressed and persecuted him.[20] The question of Kafka's family dynamics, including losses, is faced on p. 255f, and Miller well understands how fictional characters such as the family victim Gregor Samsa in "The Metamorphosis", are transformations of the author's suffering self unbeknownst to Kafka. Yet the psychobiography of Kafka is offered mainly as a vehicle for the anti-Freudian argument "that the neuroses of today were not brought about by drive deprivation or drive conflicts but by severe narcissistic traumatizations (such as humiliation, hurt feelings, sexual abuse and also by making light of childhood suffering), coupled with the necessity to repress them".[21] There is nothing wrong with making such a point but it could be greatly reinforced by research findings which would have reduced the need for polemic.

Other psychobiographies by Miller are either brief illustrative aides, such as that of Sylvia Plath's "forbidden suffering" in *For Your Own Good* (1983), or better developed but theory-bound portraits of figures begging to be heard more on their own terms. The studies of creative persons in *The Untouched Key* (1990)—Pablo Picasso, Kathe Kollwitz, Buster Keaton, Chaim Soutine and Friedrich Nietzsche—are not convincingly detailed enough to constitute "keys" to unlock the mystery of their creativity, except in the most general way. Doubters of the childhood trauma theory of creativity are likely to remain unconvinced, as when Picasso's childhood anxiety is attributed to witnessing an earthquake rather than to his fraught relations with mother and father. Miller does not begin to account for Picasso's destructive womanizing. Insights into Nietzsche's "encoded language of the child who was forbidden to express his true feelings" are of another order, but here too Nietzsche's tormented feelings about women and sexual orientation call for fuller study.[22] In the context of Bram Dijkstra's *Idols of Perversity: Fantasies of Feminine Evil in Fin-de-Siècle Culture* (1986), which studies compulsive use of Delila, Salome and other motifs of evil women, Nietzsche's preoccupations may not seem strange. But only detailed psychobiography improving upon Miller's can hope to reveal the origins of misogynistic power fantasies. Closely attuned to the collective anxieties of our time, her psychobiographical studies of demonic destructiveness, such as those of Hitler and Jurgen Bartsch in *For Your Own Good*, are the most successful. More subtle criteria are needed for individual psychobiographies of artists, writers and philosophers who shape the culture in less damaging ways.

Miller's view of creativity is virtually that of therapy itself: "The goal of therapy is to allow the once silenced child to speak and to feel".[23] Painting has limitations, being symbolic of "what was hidden in the unconscious", but it gives entry to regenerative urges and ultimately to rebirth of affirmative psychological life free of depression.[24] For all its limitations, Miller's cumulative writings on creativity put an end to the hegemony of Freudian and Kleinian theories of creativity. She opens a new era in which "anxiety situations" will be more accurately understood as the residues of childhood trauma, and creativity takes on new meaning as a natural reparative function.

Notes

1. Alice Miller, *The Drama of the Gifted Child* (1979) (New York: Basic Books, 1990), p. 25.

2. Henri F. Ellenberger, *The Discovery of the Unconscious: The History and Evolution of Dynamic Psychiatry* (London: Allen Lane, 1970). For Freud, see pp. 444–50; for Jung see pp. 669–73; summary, pp. 889–90.

3. Carl G. Jung, *Memories, Dreams and Reflections*, ed. Aniela Jaffé (New York: Vintage Books, 1965), p. 179.

4. Ibid.,p.187; Alice Miller, *Pictures of a Childhood: Sixty-six Watercolors and an Essay* (New York: Farrar, Straus and Giroux, 1986), p. 5.

5. See D.W. Winnicott, "The Squiggle Game," *Psycho-Analytic Explorations* (London: Karnac Books, 1989), pp. 299–317.

6. Alice Miller, *Pictures of a Childhood*, p. 13. Of Picasso, Miro, Klee and Chagall, Miller wrote: "their brushes were guided by the unconscious, not by neurosis"; lack of neuroses may be an unwarranted

assumption. *Thou Shalt Not Be Aware: Society's Betrayal of the Child* (New York: Meridian, 1986), p. 242.

7. Wassily Kandinsky, *Concerning the Spiritual in Art and Painting in Particular* (New York: George Wittenborn, 1955), p. 23f., p. 29. In regard to Miller's insistence on each artist finding his or her own imagery, compare Rainer Maria Rilke's *Letter to a Young Poet* (New York: W.W. Norton, 1963), pp. 18–20.

8. Paul Klee, *The Diaries, 1898–1918*, ed., Felix Klee (University of California Press, 1964), p. 3f; Will Grohman, *Paul Klee* (New York: Abrams, n.d.), p. 367. Alice Miller had read Klee's diaries: see *For Your Own Good: Hidden Cruelty in Child-Rearing and the Roots of Violence* (New York: Farrar, Straus, Giroux, 1983), p. 249.

9. Alice Miller, *Pictures of a Childhood*, p. 3. To begin painting seems to have been Miller's own decision, not directed by a therapist as in the instances of Marion Milner's patient "Susan" in *The Hands of the Living God* or Marie Naevestad's patient "Marion" in *The Colors of Rage and Love: The Process of Change in Psychotherapy Elucidated by the Patient's Own Drawings* (Oslo, Norway:Universitetsforlaget, 1979). Both Milner and Naevestad took inspiration from Melanie Klein.

10. Alice Miller, *Pictures of Childhood*, p. 3.

11. Alice Miller, *The Drama of the Gifted Child*, p. 35.

12. Jeffery M. Masson, *Final Analysis: The Making and Unmaking of a Psychoanalyst* (Reading, Mass.: Addison-Wesley, 1990), p. 179. See also Janet Malcolm, *In the Freud Archives* (New York: Vintage, 1985), pp. 50–51; 149.

13. Alice Miller, *The Drama of the Gifted Child*, p. xxi (note).

14. Alice Miller, *Banished Knowledge: Facing Childhood Injuries* (New York: Doubleday, 1990), p. 187.

15. Alice Miller, *Pictures of Childhood*, pp. 10–11, p.14.

16. Alice Miller, *Banished Knowledge*, p. 157. See Sandor Ferenczi's "Confusion of Tongues Between Adults and the Child," *International Journal of Psycho-analysis*, 30(1949): 225–230 and *The Clinical Diary of Sandor Ferenczi*, ed. J. Dupont (Harvard University Press, 1988).

17. Ibid., p. 42. See also Miller, *Thou Shalt Not Be Aware*, p. 42. for reservations about the theories of Melanie Klein and Otto Kernberg; See further, "Interview with Alice Miller," *Omni*, March, 1987, p. 80.

18. Alice Miller, *The Drama of the Gifted Child*, p. 7; *Banished Knowledge*, p. 148; *The Untouched Key: Tracing Childhood Trauma in Creativity and Destructiveness* (New York: Doubleday, 1990), p. 156; *The Drama of the Gifted Child*, "Vantage Point 1990" introduces J. Konrad Stettbacher's method of rediscovering childhood step by step, p. x.

19. Ibid., pp. 100–1, p. 111.

20. Alice Miller, *Thou Shalt Not Be Aware*, p. 242.

21. Ibid., pp. 299–300.

22. Alice Miller, *The Untouched Key*, p. 75.

23. Alice Miller, *Banished Knowledge*, p. 189.

24. Ibid., p. 163.

Part III

Creativity: The Manic-Depression Controversy

11

Nancy C. Andreasen, Kay R. Jamison and Others: Studies of Creativity

In *The Anatomy of Melancholy* (1621f) Robert Burton thought "all poets to be mad", basing his assertion on the theory of humours.[1] By "mad" Burton meant that poets were melancholic, or depressed, suffering from a predominance of black bile over the other three humours. The belief that poets and thinkers were melancholic descended to the Renaissance from Aristotle who had observed that "all those who have become eminent in philosophy or politics or poetry or the arts are clearly of an atrabilious temperament", instancing Empedocles, Socrates, and Plato.[2] Aristotle saw that excessively 'hot' or 'cold' melancholy was unproductive, while a mean temperature was likely to produce "men of genius". The Renaissance Humanist Marsilio Ficino refined Aristotle's observation about melancholia fuelling imagination and intellect. Ficino wrote in the first book of *De Vita Libri Tres* (1482-89) that adust (dried) melancholy causes mania, but natural melancholy, mixed to kindling but not burning with warmer humours, shines brightly.[3] It is interesting that this doctrine of moderate melancholic temperament as most productive in the arts should be translatable into the dysthymia and cyclothymia found in creative personalities by modern psychiatric researchers.

The theory of humoural imbalance was widely held in the Renaissance just as that of disordered neurotransmitters is now, with the refinement that the current theory is based on assaying actual brain biochemistry. A more exacting language for the same phenomena is now available; but we are almost as ignorant of the causes of disordered neurotransmitter function as were our forebears, few of whom ventured outside the humours themselves to look for causes. Ever speculative, Burton ventured causes other than being "born under Saturn" when he spoke of the melancholic having been "born of melancholy parents", a late twentieth century feature of research into childhood depressions.[4] Far-fetched though some of the commentary is, Burton was also astute in seeing melancholic temperament which "could neither be imputed to father nor mother but to his cruel nurse alone", at a time when wet nursing was common practice.[5] In the multitude of natural causes of melancholy, Burton cited "some loss, danger, death of friends", producing "sorrow and grief".[6] Presumably, he would include loss of parents, especially mother.[7] Broadly he saw fear as a cause of persistent melancholy, citing many "anxiety situations" produced by "this foul fiend of fear" and detailed at great length throughout the text.[8]

Indeed, the worst fears are of "our own parents, [who] by their offences, indiscretion, and intemperance, are our mortal enemies".[9] Here Burton clearly speaks of "anxious attachment" in the developmental process contributing to disturbed mood in later life. This cause is suggested along with genetic transmission of temperament: "That other inward, inbred cause of melancholy is our temperature, in whole or part, which we receive from our parents"; it is natural or unnatural "being an hereditary disease", Burton writes.[10] "Nature binds all creatures to love their young ones," he observes but in melancholics this love has gone badly wrong.[11] Thus for all his powerful human insights, Burton maintained the humour theory just as we do the theory of neurotransmitter malfunction. In canvassing the whole range of causes from supernatural to natural he encompassed the theory of melancholy from ancient times to his own, but he could not decide on priorities, on what causes produce what effects and in what order. The theory of humours was a safe consensus, just as the genetic disease model is a safe refuge now from difficult and disturbing psycho-social questions concerning depression as maladaptation. Burton pictures humans as subject to an array of stressors, to adversity beyond their control; his is a theory of victimhood, and he freely confesses that writing is a way of "being busy to avoid melancholy", "a kind of impostume in my head".[12] A creative scholar himself, Burton was on the track of an important causal sequence of events, but he left questions open, as we still do, because they are too emotionally charged with personal implications. Yet there can be no convincing theory of creativity without an understanding of the developmental and interpersonal meaning of depression, and depression is unlikely to be understood without greater attention to the risks of infant and child development with their effects on self-esteem. Developmental and interpersonal research are underemphasized in an era of exciting advances in neurochemical and genetic research, but they are essential if creativity is to be understood and given its rightful place in human affairs.

Recent phenomenological studies reopen the "mad poet" controversy, this time with a scientific sophistication missing in Burton's *Anatomy of Melancholy* and deficient in such later studies as those of Caesar Lombroso and Havelock Ellis.[13] The series of psychiatric studies by Nancy C. Andreasen and Kay Jamison pose the Humanities with much the same question as did Burton's in the seventeenth century: is the poet/writer merely a potential casualty of depression or is he/she a cultural leader, making discoveries that contribute to a better life for all? Burton pleaded for self-discovery and self-knowledge: "I have laid myself open - (I know it) in this treatise, turned mine inside outward: I shall be censured, I doubt not".[14] He knew reception of his book would be fickle; modern "confessional" writers and their critics take the same chance when they attempt to make sense of suicidal and other self-destructive behaviors in themselves and their subjects. Andreasen and Jamison give very little help in this regard, interpretation being not their purpose: their findings have no doubt been taken as negative and dispiriting, turning creative persons into statistical case studies. While regretting the pathologizing, and to some degree dehumanizing, of creativity their work should be welcomed.

The balance can again be tipped, reinstating a humane creativity. The argument here is that recent research in attachment theory reintroduces the humanizing element missing from strict diagnostic procedures, useful as they may be. The profiles of affective disorders and creativity will be reviewed before reframing them in attachment research findings that clarify what may be learned from the inner lives of creative persons, however disordered by anxious attachments and fear of depression.

Beginning in the 1970s, Nancy C. Andreasen showed a prevalence of bi-polar and cyclothymic disorders, rather than schizophrenia, in fiction writers. Her findings have been confirmed and elaborated by Kay Jamison and others. This turning point in theory of creativity redirects enquiry through the affective disorders, which have been the subject of intensive study. The emphasis of biological studies of affective disorders has focussed on their genetic transmission and on biochemical abnormalities in neurotransmitters regulating mood. The gain of knowledge has been rapid and exciting, but not without premature conclusions and distortion of the field of questioning.[15] These studies of creativity reflect the research bias that pushes aside questions of motivation and meaning in favor of mechanism. Little place has been left for developmental studies, and nothing is said by Andreasen or Jamison about depression and quality of early infant-mother attachment. (John Bowlby's major studies of maternal loss and depression only began being published in the 1960s, although these early studies do not bear directly on bipolar pathology.) Because developmental theories are neglected in deference to a range of genetically "fated" neurochemical disorders, there can be no compensating adaptive or "reparative" function in their theory of creativity. It therefore seems to put down the arts as humanity's finest achievement, raising up a scientific methodology of limited applicability and certainly without capacity to explain the creative impulse.

There was clear justification for Andreasen's initial studies. A literary scholar turned psychiatrist, she was worried by the high suicide rate among leading American poets such as Robert Lowell, Sylvia Plath and Anne Sexton which appeared to be symptomatic of something unhealthy in the cultural climate of the 1960s and 1970s. Indeed critics such as A. Alvarez publicized what they called "extremist" poetry glorifying self-violence. A mental health professional might well be concerned, but the study of poets was not open to her. Instead, Andreasen and her colleagues set up the most methodically exacting study of fiction writers ever attempted. They studied fifteen leading figures in the Iowa Writer's Workshop, looking for psychiatric symptoms. Expecting a prevalence of schizophrenia in self-destructive creative people, instead they found affective disorders—mainly bipolar or manic-depressive—in a high proportion of the subjects. This should not have been surprising as there had been experimental foreshadowings of psychopathology in creative people. For instance, in 1962 D. W. MacKinnon had reported a MMPI (Minnesota Multiphasic Personality Inventory) study of architects that revealed a prevalence of psychopathology but also of adequate control mechanisms.[16] Nonetheless, the impact of Andreasen's 1974 study was profound and lasting. A popular journal *Psychology Today* reported under the heading "Creativity and the Troubled Mind" that Andreasen's extended studies had revealed that eighty percent of the writer group, in contrast to thirty percent of controls, had been treated for mood disorders. Forty three percent of writers showed some degree of manic-depressive illness, in comparison with ten percent of the others. Alcoholism afflicted many writers and two of the expanded group of thirty had taken their lives—dramatic testimony of the danger with which creative people live.[17]

Nancy Andreasen published her findings widely over more than a ten-year span, examining new facets of bipolar disorder and creativity. Her position is clearly stated in "Suffering in Art": "Creative writers are the torchbearers of civilization. In recent years many have been unable to complete their marathon. The torch they carried was their art, not their lives. It will advance civilization only to the extent that it sheds the light of sanity rather than insanity."[18] But there is very little in her scientific studies to show what "sanity" might be, or where to look for it; nor is she eager to examine the lives of creative persons. Her studies powerfully reinforce the writer's psychopathology rather than potential for health and sanity. For instance, "Creativity and Psychosis" notes that the conceptual style of writers resembles "mania more than schizophrenia and . . . if overinclusiveness is an index of thought disorder, manics may have a more florid thought disorder than schizophrenics".[19]

To Andreasen family studies do not mean studying family dynamics predisposing to bipolar disorder but lines of probable genetic transmission of the disorder. In "The Creative Writer: Psychiatric Symptoms and Family History" she found "a striking prevalence of psychiatric disorder in general among the primary relatives of the writers compared with the controls".[20] While admitting to the presence of high anxiety among writers, she puts "the extent to which the writers struggled with despair and its effects upon their work . . . outside the scope of this paper" and never really addresses it.[21] This was an opportunity missed as she seemed about to identify "anxious attachment" as pathogenic. The genetic assumption goes unexamined, whereas there is ample evidence that family dynamics play a large part in cyclothymic mood disorders characteristic of creative persons. In "'Genius and Insanity' Revisited: Psychiatric Symptoms and Family History in Creative Writers" Andreasen and Canter reaffirm that family pattern tends "toward the development of both creativity and illness", allowing that many writers "described subjective feelings of unhappiness or trauma in their early lives".[22] Yet they say that writers and controls did not differ significantly in early childhood experiences and that although "a somewhat greater number of writers than controls described their relationship with their parents as poor", they saw "no effect either on the development of creativity or on psychiatric disorder in the writers and perhaps even that genetic factors may be of primary importance".[23] Clearly a more sensitive instrument was needed to discover the presence of anxieties regarding parenting so that attempts could be made to link these anxieties with thematic concerns in the writing. We will see that there is now such an instrument in the Adult Attachment Interview (AAI), devised by the psychologist Mary Main.

Andreasen never broke out of a strictly genetic causality, even lacking the research to back up the general point that, assuming a genetic etiology for bipolar disorder, this hypothesis has never been proven. In 1980 she wrote starkly: "creativity and mood disorder tend to run together in families", and in 1987 she again reported "that the families of the writers were riddled with both creativity and mental illness, while in the families of the control subjects much of the illness and creativity seemed to be randomly scattered".[24] Thus for all her concern with the self-destructiveness of writers, Andreasen does not address questions of family and social development strongly implied in her material. While science sharpens up her diagnostic findings, it blunts the general point she was hoping to make, and it prevents any suggestion that creativity might be healthily adaptive in conditions of emotional distress.

It is a long step from John E. Drevdahl and Raymond B. Cattell's "Personality and Creativity in Artists and Writers" (1958) which found their subjects to have "divine discontent" while "emotionally mature" and not evidently cyclothymic, to Ruth L. Richards's careful study in 1981 confirming the1974 findings of Andreasen and Canter of high levels of active and personality disorder in their subjects.[25] While noting drawbacks in Andreasen and Canter's study—lack of a random sample and all male subjects—Richards accepted their findings as "a mixed picture of adaptive and apparently maladaptive personality traits". She saw the need for further study of a creativity psychopathology relationship, in some cases probably genetic in origin.[26] This was a reasonable position to take but the next development, in studies of manic depression in creative persons by Kay Jamison, took matters to an unexpected extreme.

Unlike Andreasen, Jamison offers biographical studies of creative persons, but they are highly selective and presuppose genetically caused, and neurochemically mediated, bipolar disorder. Jamison is not a literary critic trained to examine the thematic subtleties of texts but a psychologist with a particular mind set. She assembles her cases to illustrate the predominance of bipolar disorder in creative persons, perhaps because she herself has been a bipolar sufferer. Maintained on lithium, Jamison courageously published her experience of manic depression in *An Unquiet Mind: A Memoir of Moods and Madness* (1996). Understandably, she wants her illness to be seen as having a genetic origin, writing: "It is an illness that is biological in its origin, yet one that feels psychological in the experience of it; an illness that is unique in conferring advantage and pleasure, yet one that brings in its wake almost unendurable suffering and, not infrequently, suicide".[27] Having once attempted suicide herself, Jamison recreates as much of her emotional history as she is able, but family interaction essential to know about is scanted, and possible sources of childhood anxiety and fright are not revealed. We know that beneath the genetic dogma there is a human story as Jamison is so deeply concerned with the healing power of love. Yet her narrative is crafted to say less than it seems to say about childhood stressors and their reanimation in adult relationships. To secure the credibility of genetic determinism, Jamison has searched through literary history to find as much supporting evidence as possible, with impressive but distorting results.

Jamison's fullest psychobiography is of the flamboyant and disorderly English Romantic poet Lord Byron, who by his own estimate was afflicted by bad genetic inheritance. Jamison's assessment of Byron's disastrous relational life is a triumph of nature over nurture: a study in genetic determinism, neglecting attention to pathogenic factors in his development. Born with a deformed foot, Byron spent his youth rebelliously proving himself by various exploits. But physical deformity was exacerbated by loss of father at age three and domination by a temperamental mother. Byron is reported to have had both "a predisposition to grief" and a love-hate relationship with his tyrannical mother.[28] Byron complained as an adult of his mother: "Her temper is too variable, and when inflamed, so furious, that I dread our meeting . . . ".[29] What must it have been to be a child of this woman, however buffered by the paid caretakers usual in the upper class? There is no room in Jamison's theory for the anxious attachment of the child Byron and his blatantly Jocasta mother. His promiscuity, probable bisexuality, incest with a half sister and general capriciousness cannot be explained by inherited temperament alone. Perhaps they can never be fully explained, any more than his poetic sensitivity to language and imagery; but a skillful psychobiographer could build a case more grounded in developmental studies than is Jamison's. It would be a case respectful of Byron's own insight into his excesses and of his capacity for repairing the damage, if only on the aesthetic plane.

Jamison's biographical sketches of bipolar poets and composers in chapter 13 of *Manic Depressive Illness* is perfunctory. Her prejudged selected cases eliminate the important early loss of a parent variable, as with the poets William Cowper, Samuel Taylor Coleridge and Edgar Allen Poe. Traumatic, anxiety-causing childhood events are not considered, even though in the same book Goodwin and Jamison discuss how "precipitating events play an important role in the onset of the first few episodes" of bipolar illness, however unmotivated later episodes may seem to be.[30] More telling for her argument is Table 14.2, a "partial listing of major 20th century American poets born between 1895 and 1935 with documented histories of manic-depressive illness" in which five of the eight poets took their lives.[31] The suicides are associated with severe mood swings, but nothing is said of underlying, developmental causes of despair traceable to lost or disharmonious attachments to parents. Jamison speaks of creative persons "learning through intense and deep emotional experiences" and of how "Pain's dominion fills novels, biographies and autobiographies . . . " but never examines them in detailed relational terms as reputable psychobiographers must do.[32] Figure 14-3 (p. 353) shows her 1989 sample of British writers and artists to be suffering more from depressive illness than from bipolar disorder, despite the poets where bipolarity is elevated. Thus another look is needed—outside of the undoubted genetic vulnerability of some persons—for probable sources of reactive and other non-cycling depressions, or for depressions whose cycling is undramatic.

Jamison's mission is to show the rewards of bipolar disorder while de-emphasizing the underlying anxiety and despair of relational origin.[33] The high suicide rate symptomatic of a culture in crisis is avoided as it points to complicated and unsettling psycho-social questions. "Clouds and Silver Linings: Positive Experiences Associated with Primary Affective Disorder" (1980) notes that "More than ninety percent of the total sample reported a perceived increase in overall sensitivity as a result of having a mood disorder", and their creativity was so enhanced that the manic phase became almost addictive.[34] In 1989, Jamison reported on "Mood Disorders and

Patterns of Creativity in British Writers and Artists" a study of hypomania and creativity finding "that the milder forms of hypomania may represent the more productive phases of affective illness."[35] Thus she moderated her views toward those of Hagop Akiskal and Ruth Richards who see creativity associated with milder forms of depression such as cyclothymia or, as Richards put it: creativity is enhanced in subjects showing "perhaps 'subclinical' expressions of potential bipolar liability". [36]

The British psychiatrist Felix Post confirmed in "Creativity and Psychopathology" (1994) Andreasen's and Jamison's main findings. Starting with a wide-ranging selection of 291 world famous men studied from their biographies, he found that "severe personality deviations were unduly frequent only in the case of visual artists and writers", by which he meant a prevalence of affective disorders.[37] Post's findings of seventy-two percent depressions in writers independently confirmed Andreasen's figure of eighty percent in the Iowa writers' workshop group—a figure more than doubling depressions among scientists, artists, intellectuals, politicians and composers.[38] Post's findings differ mainly in severity of affective disorder although he does not comment directly on incidence of bipolarity. Using DSM criteria, writers, artists and marginally intellectuals were found to have more "seriously disabling and disruptive personality deviations than the general public.[39] While varying in some details with Jamison's findings of hypomania in creative writers, he had no basic disagreement.

Working on a broader scale of psychopathology, Post found "ninety percent of the creative writers exhibited some traits of DSM personality disorders, and in twenty percent these had been seriously disruptive"[40] He found mainly avoidant, obsessive-compulsive and dependent personalities in his sample of writers, with depression incidental to these other diagnoses. As noted, severe depressions were commonest among novelists and playwrights and least so among artists. Suicide rates in Post's sample were not unduly high, unlike that among American poets studied by Jamison. Surprisingly, anxiety levels were not found to be elevated as anxiety and depression are usually linked. This finding may result from limitations of Post's method of gathering information from biographies. He worked alone and did not do content analyses of writers' productions to discover what their thematic preoccupations actually were. He did, however, note of writers that "regardless of the blocks and breakdowns which many had suffered, they were powerfully driven by the urge to create"—close to suggesting a reparative urge.[41]

Whereas Andreasen's 1974 studies asserted that her creative subjects came from stable families, and that early environment was not in question, Post is not so sure. Not a genetic determinist, he comments: "Fifty-six percent of writers, the category with the highest prevalence of psychopathology, had unhappy childhoods, as against twenty-six percent of thinkers and, least often, ten percent of composers".[42] As to clustering of psychopathology in the families of creative persons, first described in a German study by Juda, Post keeps an open mind. He does not say just what "unhappy childhood" means and proposes more studies to find out. Familial influences, including study of developmental styles and family interactions are indicated, together with the genesis of bipolar disorder among the varieties of depression.

Biographical studies of emotional disorder in writers are presented by Gordon Claridge, Ruth Pryor and Gwen Watkins in *Sounds From the Bell Jar* (1990). Claridge is a psychologist expert in current psychiatric diagnostic criteria, while his co-authors are literary scholars who assemble the biographical data for him to assess. Before the DSM gained authority, such an exercise would have been unthinkable, as would Post's; together they reinforce the pathologization of creativity, earlier adduced by Andreasen and Jamison from their findings of prevalent bipolar disorder. Indeed Claridge's subjects—such as Christopher Smart, William Cowper, John Ruskin, A.C. Benson, Virginia Woolf and Sylvia Plath—are labelled psychotic, with far worse outcomes than most in Andreasen's sample. This group is said to be both abnormally "skinless" against life's hurts, yet intensely imaginative, the outcomes tragic with little evidence of healing. Nonetheless, this does not obviate the presence of a self-healing impulse in each of the subjects, evidenced by their determination to rework for greater clarity the anxious attachments of formative years.

Claridge is eager to show familial transmissions of emotional disorder, as in the case of A.C. Benson's insanity which had "a strong endogenous, biological component", easily activated by losses.[43] Family pathology is indeed Claridge's theme, yet he is too informed (as the biographical profiles show) to assert simple biological causality as Jamison tries to do. "These facts of inheritance are no explanation of psychoses, but they do point to some trait or traits of vulnerability, the expression of which was shaped by the experiences and circumstances of our subjects' lives"[44] Early parental loss, and other stressful attachments, are mentioned, yet Claridge seems unaware of how attachment theory would help to remove the terrible fatedness of his theory of creativity. Without recognizing an inherent reparative urge, however thwarted, creative writing remains a mere illustration of psychiatry's new ability to categorize psychopathology.

A better understanding is needed of the developmental and interpersonal meaning of depression. Genetic determinism oversimplifies and dehumanizes the complicated aetiologies of depressions. Bipolar depressions probably have a discoverable genetic predisposition, but it remains to be located in the chromosomes. Monopolar reactive depressions are less genetically determined, and circumstantial causes are generally looked for. In both it can be argued that pathological biochemical changes are the result of learned styles of reacting to high stress, especially during childhood. Attachment theory has a place for genetically based biochemical predisposition to depression, but its emphasis is quite different from that found in the work of Andreasen, Jamison and Claridge.[45] Attachment theory calls for a revised protocol in the psychobiography of depressives. A reliable psychobiography of a creative person with depression must take into account: (a) sensitivity factors (b) vulnerability factors and (c) provoking factors for the depressiveness which creativity attempts to contact and heal. Sensitivity factors concern genetic and familial transmissions of "permission" to become manic or depressed under certain interpersonal conditions. Early loss of a parent, or parents, greatly increases the risk of depression when there is a traumatic provoking agent. Vulnerability factors are lack of close sustaining relationships, including troubled sexuality, lack of employment, having dependent children or elders etc. Provoking agents are crises, or events interpreted as such, for which normal coping strategies are not available. Provoking agents upset the precarious balance in persons temperamentally and genetically disposed to depression, who for social reasons are poorly integrated into the community. Low self-esteem and cruel twists of fate assail a poorly integrated personality, leaving mood change, depression or mania, or both, its only option. Thus consideration of heredity, development and current experience is needed in assessing liability to depression and the quality of creative response. Informed judgment is needed to see the relationship among factors predisposing to depression when considering the meaning of creativity. Review of some neglected studies will help to illustrate how sensitivity, vulnerability and provocations to depression may operate.[46]

In the psychobiography of creative persons where depression is present, the sequence sensitivity, vulnerability and provoking agents is followed by symptom formation and response. The creative response addresses the discomposure and pain of symptoms and may take the form of artistic creativity. Creativity is the positive feature of some psychopathology and, to be seen as more than an epiphenomenon, a thoroughgoing developmental sequence is needed. There are few reliable guides taking us beyond "biological" determinism into the psycho-social factors with which biological "sensitivity" must be associated to produce cyclothymia or manic-depressive disorder.

The path breaking study by Mabel Blake Cohen et al., "An Intensive Study of Twelve Cases of Manic Depressive Psychoses", together with two elaborating studies by Robert W. Gibson and others, made a start. Of course, the family dynamics proposed in these studies need reconsideration in the light of improved understanding of attachment, especially abusive types of attachment. But Cohen's and Gibson's insistence on observing real-life interactions with bipolar disorder as a pathological adaptation to demands on the sufferer, is exemplary. Although difficult, their studies could be redesigned in contemporary terms.

To summarize their findings, Cohen proposed a family configuration for the future bipolar sufferer in which the family was isolated, "different" from the community which it aspired to join. The difference might be ethnic or due to ostracism, with the father usually held by the mother to be weak and ineffectual—the cause of isolation. Initially, a caring attentive parent, the mother singled out a promising boy or girl to "push" toward delivering the family from its obscurity. The delegated child was to establish or restore family prestige by outstanding accomplishment. To achieve this, the once-caring mother had disciplined her chosen child's independent rebelliousness from an early age so as to insure conformity to community standards. Thus, from the child's point of view, her caring inexplicably turned to harsher discipline, setting up what Gibson describes as intense anxiety preventing the child from "integrating his concepts of the good mother and bad mother into a single person."[47] This anticipates what Bowlby and others describe as "anxious attachment"of the anxious-avoidant type. Gibson emphasizes changed mothering styles more than does Cohen in accounting for the bipolar dynamic.

He agrees with Cohen that intense "dependency" is engendered and kept out of awareness, along with envy arising from the wish to excel. The future bipolar sufferer is thus kept unaware of what he or she actually feels, being delegated to perform a task for the mother rather than realizing a self in the normal way. Driven by envy arising from implicit instructions to compete with others, the child "undersells" him- or herself in order to protectively ingratiate and monopolize gains. A spurious sense of charming harmlessness masks the desperate will to dominate. A hypomanic presentation of self develops, with true reciprocity less in evidence than a sterotyped social performance. Self-absorbed, the hypomanic youth, being out of touch with his or her own feelings, cannot contact feelings of others and so remains unmodified by them. A kind of narcissism surrounds anxiety over success, and a manipulative style with others is the result. Manipulation by ingratiating behavior, rather than outright obsessional control, is characteristic, although obsessiveness in performing tasks may be evident.[48] The self-awareness attributed by Patricia Crittenden to the Creative A/C (defended and coercive) personality type is comparatively lacking in the hypomanics who fend off risk of depression.

Failure to contact and accept depressive affect as an essential constituent of life reduces creativity. It also reduces empathy and the possibility of enriched reciprocal relationships. The result of unreciprocated "dependency needs" is emptiness and unassuaged anxiety about abandonment. While energetically driven and seemingly alive, the hypomanic personality style is dangerously empty and unreactive, a false self organization given to manic attacks and ingratiating expiations to forestall depression. As Cohen comments: "Thus, the process of underselling both for the sake of denying envy and in order to become the recipient of gifts from the other, often reaches the point where these persons actually paralyze the use of their own endowments and creative abilities"[49] Gibson further comments that "it is doubtful that genetic and biological factors could so influence the development of interpersonal relations as to account for the remarkably consistent dynamic descriptions of the personalities of these patients".[50] The Cohen-Gibson psychogenic theory of bipolar disorder has bearings on creativity that need testing in view of Andreasen's and Jamison's assertions. Clearly, there is a limited range of bipolar adaptation which is sufficiently open and flexible to be attracted to the arts and called "creative". This range needs accurate description and study in actual examples in the lives of persons who used artistic creativity to overcome early developmental deficits.

Notes

1. Robert Burton, *The Anatomy of Melancholy*, ed. H. Jackson (London: J. M. Dent, 1961), vol.1, p. 112.

2. Quoted in Lawrence Babb, *The Elizabethan Malady: A Study of Melancholia in English Literature from 1580–1642* (East Lansing: Michigan State University Press, 1951), p. 59.

3. Ibid., p. 60.

4. Burton, *The Anatomy of Melancholy*, vol. 1, p, 172. Burton also recognized the adverse effect for infants of having "a melancholy mother" (vol. 1, 212) and approvingly quotes Pliny on the adverse consequences of swaddling: "For to begin at the hour of his birth ... he is born naked, and falls a-whining at the very first, he is swaddled and bound up like a prisoner, cannot help himself, and so he continues to life's end" (vol. 1, p. 272) Burton thought that "children live in a perpetual slavery" (vol. 1, p. 278).

5. Burton, *Anatomy of Melancholy*, vol. 1, p. 331. Persecution by witch-like women and bad wives is also a theme of Burton's: see vol. 1, p.109 and p. 253.

6. Ibid., vol. 1, p. 279; see also vol.1, p. 275; p. 386; pp. 389–90.

7. See John Bowlby, "The Origins of Attachment Theory," in *A Secure Base: Clinical Applications of Attachment Theory* (London: Routledge, 1988).

8. Burton, *Anatomy of Melancholy*, vol. 1, p. 261; See also vol.1, p. 286.

9. Ibid., vol. 1, p. 135; see also vol. 1, p.135, vol. 3, p. 23.

10. Ibid., vol. 1, p. 211.

11. Ibid., vol. 3, p. 31.

12. Ibid., vol. 1, pp. 20–21.

13. Cesare Lombroso, *The Man of Genius* (London: Walter Scott, 1891); Havelock Ellis, *A Study of British Genius* (London: Hurst and Blackett, 1904).

14. Burton, *Anatomy of Melancholy*, vol. 1, p. 27.

15. See discussion by Leo Cytryn, M.D. and Donald H. McKnew M.D. in *Growing Up Sad: Childhood Depression and Its Treatment* (New York: W. W. Norton, 1996), p. 174f.

16. D.W. Mackinnon, "The Personality Correlates of Creativity: A Study of American Architects," *Creativity: Selected Readings*, ed. P. E. Vernon (Harmondsworth: Penguin, 1970), p. 307.

17. Constance Holden, "Creativity and the Troubled Mind," *Psychology Today*, April, 1987, pp. 9–10.

18. Nancy Andreasen, "Suffering and Art," in *The Healing Arts in Dialogue*, ed. U. Trautmann (Carbondale: Southern Illinois Press, 1981), pp. 38 –9.

19. Nancy Andreasen and Pauline Powers, "Creativity and Psychosis: An Examination of Conceptual Style," *Archives of General Psychiatry*, 32 (1975):70.

20. Nancy Andreasen and Arthur Canter, "The Creative Writer: Psychiatric Symptoms and Family History," *Comprehensive Psychiatry*, 15, no. 2 (1974): 126.

21. Ibid., pp. 128–29.

22. Nancy Andreasen and Arthur Canter, "'Genius and Insanity' Revisited: Psychiatric Symptoms and Family History in Creative Writers," *Life*

History Research in Psychopathology, ed. R. Wirt et al. (Minneapolis: University of Minnesota Press, 1974), pp. 197, 198.

23. Ibid., pp. 199–200.

24. Nancy Andreasen, "Mania and Creativity," *Mania an Evolving Concept*, ed. R. H. Belmaker and H. M. van Praag (SP Medical & Scientific Books, 1980), p. 385; "Creativity and Mental Illness: Prevalence Rates in Writers and Their First-Degree Relatives," *American Journal of Psychiatry*, 144 (1987):1290.

25. John E. Drevdahl and Raymond B. Cattell, "Personality and Creativity in Artists and Writers," *Journal of Clinical Psychology*, 14 (1958).

26. Ruth L. Richards, "Relationships Between Creativity and Psychopathology: An Evaluation and Interpretation of the Evidence," *Genetic Psychology Monographs* (Harvard Medical School) no.103 (1981): 294–5, 317.

Methodology has been criticized in the work of Nancy Andreasen and later, Kay R. Jamison. Albert Rothenberg sees a rush to affirm bipolarity in creative persons, noting that because Andreasen "clearly knew who in her study were writers and who were controls and was at the same time assessing her own hypotheses, some conscious or unconscious bias inevitably must have operated" (*Creativity and Madness: New Findings and Old Stereotypes* (Baltimore: The Johns Hopkins University Press, 1990) p.150). Further, "the criteria for creativity and for choosing controls were inexplicit and misleading" (ibid. p.151).

In the case of Jamison's treatment of British writers, "no attempt at independent diagnostic assessment was made" and non-creative controls were missing from the study. (ibid. pp. 151–52). Although Rothenberg does not consider studies by Andreasen (1975f) and Jamison (1989) to be valid, he affirms the redirection they give the study of creativity, mood disorders and affective illnesses (ibid., p. 153).

In "Are Creative Writers Mad?" Martin S. Lindauer states that "If there is a link between writers and pathology, it has not been proven" (*Dionysus in Literature: Essays on Literary Madness*, ed. B.

M. Rieger (Bowling Green, OH: Bowling Green State University, Popular Press, 1994, p. 42.). Lindauer asserts that "creative persons as a group are healthy" (ibid., p. 37), and that he doubts all studies to the contrary. While allowing that "Andreasen's study of the mental health of writers is a solid empirical achievement" (ibid., p. 39), Lindauer proposes a more rigorous set of procedures to improve the sampling method, the control group, the measures used, justification for generalization and alternative explanations. He admits that Andreasen's findings have been highly influential and are reinforced by Kay Jamison's, which he had not seen at the time of writing.

Rothenberg and Lindauer make little of Adèle Juda's pioneering "The Relationship Between Highest Mental Capacity and Psychic Abnormalities," *The American Journal of Psychiatry*, 106, no. 1–12 (1949–50) : 296f , which first detected by statistics the possibility of manic depressive disorder and cyclothymia in creative persons. Whereas Juda found about two-thirds of her sample of architects, sculptors, painters, musicians and poets to be "psychically normal", she found "psychoneurosis" to affect the remaining one-third (p. 298); the most "psychopaths" were among poets and composers. Juda's terminology such as finding "schizoid eccentrics" (or "schizothymic constitution") in all groups lacks clarity, but she was the first to see manic-depression rather than schizophrenia as important to the study of creativity.

A prevalence of bipolar mood change, combined with high talent, in creativity is argued by H. S. Akiskal and K. Akiskal in "Reassessing the Prevalence of Bipolar Disorders: Clinical Significance and Artistic Creativity *Psychiatrie et Psychobiographie*, 3 (1988). Following Juda's remarks (see above, p. 298), the Akiskals "suggest that repeated self-doubt that comes with recurrent depression is an important ingredient of creativity, but because original ideas or artistic forms are often initially rejected, the self-confidence that comes with repeated bouts of hypomania can help in rehearsing these ideas or artistic forms until they are either perfected or accepted by society" (p. 345).

27. Kay Redfield Jamison, *An Unquiet Mind* (New York: Alfred A. Knopf, 1995) p. 6. Her friend Frances Lear, also a bi-polar sufferer, calls Jamison "part intellectual, part visionary, part warrior, she will remove

the stigma from mental illness" (*The Second Seduction* (New York: Alfred A. Knopf, 1992), p. 176).

28. Kay Redfield Jamison, *Touched with Fire: Manic Depressive Illness and the Artistic Temperament* (New York: The Free Press, 1993), p. 153. Byron's most recent biographer, Phyllis Grosskurth, accepts without challenge Jamison's deterministic account of Byron's manic-depression, showing how easily such opinion is taken as fact (*Byron: The Flawed Angel* (Toronto: Macfarlane Walter & Ross, 1997), pp. 56–57).

29. Ibid., p. 160. Remarking on "excesses of psychoanalytic speculation, along with other abuses of psychobiography" (p. 3), Jamison cautions about diagnoses by biographers (pp. 57, 59). She does not question that genetically transmitted liability to emotional disorder might also risk reductionism.

30. Fredrick K. Goodwin and Kay R. Jamison, *Manic-Depressive Illness* (New York: Oxford University Press, 1990), p. 142.

31. Ibid., p. 347.

32. Ibid., p. 341.

33. See Ibid., pp. 354–55.

34. Kay Jamison, "Clouds and Silver Linings: Positive Experiences Associated with Primary Affective Disorders," *American Journal of Psychiatry*, 137, no. 2 (1980): 200–1.

35. Kay Jamison, "Mood Disorders and Patterns of Creativity in British Writers and Artists," *Psychiatry*, 52 (1989): 131–32.

36. C.H., "Manic Depression and Creativity," *Science*, 233 (1986): 725. Cyclothymia has long been recognized as frequent among creative people; see Russell Brain, *Some Reflections on Genius and Other Essays* (London: Pitman, 1960), pp. 20–21.

37. Felix Post, "Creativity and Psychopathology: A Study of 291 World-Famous Men," *British Journal of Psychiatry*, 165 (1994): 22

38. Ibid., p. 32.

39. Ibid., p. 32. An experienced clinician, Post claims that his DSM-III-R diagnoses are made with "some confidence" (p. 24).

40. Ibid., p. 27.

41. Ibid., p. 31.

42. Ibid., p. 24.

43. Gordon Claridge et al., *Sounds From the Bell Jar: Ten Psychotic Authors* (London: Macmillan, 1990), p. 180. See p. 227 for the Benson genogram.

44. Ibid., p. 229.

45. See John Bowlby, *Loss, Sadness and Depression*, vol.3 of *Attachment and Loss* (London, The Hogarth Press, 1980), p. 261f, for discussion of endocrine changes in infant primates and humans following high stress as in separation and loss of mother. For attempts to close the profound gulf between biological and psychodynamic studies of emotional disorder, see Allan N. Schore, *Affect Regulation and the Origin of the Self: The Neurobiology Emotional Development*, pp. 405–417. For Schore, as for Bowlby, stressful environmental events are believed to precede adverse neurochemical changes. Schore writes: "The inability to adapt to stress and the continued activation or inhibition of internal systems that is inappropriate to a particular environmental situation essentially defines all psychiatric disorders. I believe that every type of early forming primitive disorder involves, to some extent, altered orbital prefrontal function." He continues: "The dynamic capacities and limitations of ... a reparative system are forged in early dyadic interactive repair transactions that induce transitions out of disruptive states of affective distress. In situations where the caregiver routinely does not participate in reparative functions, the resulting unmodulated psychobiological dysregulation reflects a dysregulated brain chemistry" (p. 413).

46. See George W. Brown and Tirril Harris, *Social Origins of Depression: A Study of Psychiatric Disorder* (New York: The Free Press, 1978), chapter 16; chart, p. 265.

47. Robert W. Gibson, Mabel B. Cohen, and Robert A. Cohen, " On the Dynamics of the Manic Depressive Personality," *American Journal of Psychiatry*, 115 (1959):1102.

48. Frederick Goodwin and Kay Jamison give obsessions low value among cognitive and perceptual symptoms of bi-polar disorder, but their criteria are not discussed. See table 2.5 in *Manic-Depressive Illness*, p. 43.

49. Mabel Blake Cohen et al., "An Intensive Study of Twelve Cases of Manic-Depressive Psychosis," *Psychiatry*, 17 (1954): 120. Elaboration on the dynamics of early attachment in future manic-depressive sufferers is offered by Silvano Arieti MD and Jules Bemporad MD in *Severe and Mild Depression: The Psychotherapeutic Approach* (New York: Basic Books, 1978), pp. 130–37.

50. Robert Gibson et al., "On the Dynamics of the Manic-Depressive Personality," p. 1106.

12

Three Bipolar Poets Reconsidered: Robert Lowell, Anne Sexton and Sylvia Plath

Employing the Cohen-Gibson hypothesis in biographical consideration of three bipolar poets is revealing. The confessional poets Robert Lowell, Anne Sexton and Sylvia Plath show a fit between anxiety-ridden developmental experiences—infant and childhood stressors at the level of trauma—and corrective creative endeavor through poetry. Extensive biographical materials are available for each of these poets, from which salient features will be derived. The poets knew each other and were mutually influencing in their daring pursuit of self-revelation. They perhaps never saw, however, the commonality of formative experience and character structure that explains their use of the creative impulse to face down manic-depressive tendencies. The ordered poem is a place of sanctuary where fierce emotions are recognized but withheld from action. It is a necessary testing ground for feelings not acted upon of rage and calm that need understanding if life is to be manageable. That these self-destructive poets finally did not understand themselves does not invalidate the attempts to do so. By saying the tabooed, the unsayable, they broke into new territory which can only be mapped by the insights of dynamic psychiatry.

While Robert Lowell's life (1917–1977) and art conform most closely to the Cohen-Gibson theory, those of Anne Sexton and Sylvia Plath are good matches. The creativity of each can scarcely be understood apart from formative life events, from anxiety over an abusive, weak or absent father to an over-controlling mother. Each poet exhausted his or her repertoire of adaptations, including that of poetic creativity, ending their lives violently. It is well known that Sexton and Plath suicided, while Lowell died of a heart attack which his biographer Ian Hamilton calls "a suicide wish".[1] Lowell's pensive sadness is noted by Hamilton as characteristic: "for him the whole act of remembering was full of sadness, sadness for what had been lost—not just to memory, but lost".[2] Legendary for unpredictability, Lowell had intimidated friends and lost lovers by manic misbehavior. But behind the excesses was intense awareness of the losses in his family history. The probing sensitivity of such poems in *Life Studies* as "My Last Afternoon with Uncle Devereux Winslow" and "Commander Lowell, 1887–1950", his father, bring order and proportion to recollections. By reconstructing his family, Lowell tried to see himself as sufferer and agent of suffering. He needed steadying reference points —especially in male figures— to counter his terrifying tendency to disintegrate. The most telling poem about his mother concerns accompanying her corpse home from Italy in 1954. Another, "During Fever", tries to see her personal history synoptically. These are affecting poems from a sensibility attuned to experience, no doubt, by psychotherapy. The insights are as sensitive as could be wished, yet (before lithium) Lowell could swerve dangerously into what he called "the old menacing hilarity" accompanied by outbursts of violence.[3] To quote Lowell, there would follow "the usual somberness after mania, jaundice of the spirit."[4]

The essentials of Lowell's background are as follows: a product of distinguished Boston families, Robert's father combined "a weak character and strong lineage", while his ambitious wife Charlotte Winslow had a "natural bossiness" driving her wish to assert social prominence.[5] His father's career as a naval officer caused the family to lead a nomadic existence until settling back in Boston at his wife's insistence. Scion of a lesser branch of the Lowells, the elder Robert was by no means assured of a place in society. Conformity to navy regulations by the father and the social code insisted upon by his wife impressed the son, their only child who often felt himself a rebel. Thus the family of three was an isolate aspiring to enter the ranks of a closed upper class, with Charlotte urgently in the lead but despairing of her weak husband's fitness for the task. Attention was thus directed onto son Robert who was first expected to excel at school and then in Harvard University—which he did but at risk of meeting maternal wishes rather than his own. Meanwhile his father was in decline, having unsuccessfully entered business after being persuaded by Charlotte to leave the navy. By nagging him into conformity with her wishes she left him "in his son's eyes, a ruined man, emasculated: 'In his forties, Father's soul went underground' ", as Hamilton reports Robert's comment. [6]

Cohen and Gibson's point about the mother of bipolar sufferers having changed attitudes early in development is well documented. At first "I was a little doll in a white sailor suit"; "But when I was at least three years old all that began to change. I could no longer see my mother as that rarely present, transfigured, Sunday-best version of my nurse. I saw her as my mother, as a rod, or a scolding, rusty hinge—as a human being". As Hamilton phrases it, Robert was 'enthralled' by her: "From a tender age, Lowell became a keen student of enslavement. And from his father he learned that decency and good intentions can be abject".[7] An observer commented that Charlotte disapproved of her son: "he was so clumsy, so sloppy, so ill-mannered ... I really think there was a psychological fixation on dominating Cal [Robert's nickname] by that woman. And what does a child do—with an obsessed mother and a weak father who goes along with that obsession?"[8]

Similar considerations arise in the life and art of Anne Sexton (1928-74), who studied poetry with Lowell at Boston University. The Cohen-Gibson psychogenic theory of bipolar disorder also illuminates her startlingly personal poetry, a release which no doubt prolonged and improved her life but failed to prevent suicide. Sexton's history of chronically insecure attachments was diagnostically labelled everything from "hysteric" to "schizophrenic", but depression with marked bipolarity is the best description of what she suffered.

Anne Sexton was introduced to poetry in her therapy with a remarkable psychiatrist, Dr. Martin Orne. That Sexton was a "difficult" patient who had attempted suicide, Orne's tapes, released to her biographer, disclosed. Whereas Anne thought she could only be good as a prostitute to make men feel sexually powerful, Dr. Orne found a way to better gratification through her creative unconscious. Dr. Orne may not have followed Sexton right to the source of her feelings of self-disgust and meaninglessness, but he did open the way. Through therapy enlightened by increasingly adept poetry writing, a kind of meaning for Anne's formative experiences was constructed. As these were pre-attachment theory days, the terms were none too precise, and Dr. Orne may not have grasped the full construct presented by Anne's life and art. Nonetheless, the flood of poems beginning in 1956/7 owed much to perceptiveness about his patient. "Poems don't lie", she said: "the difference between confession and poetry, is, after all art".[9] Poetry and therapy 'interlocked', making Dr. Orne's task easier. When he moved from Boston to Philadelphia, Anne wrote of her distressed reaction: "I'm not (overtly) depressed . . . oh no MANIC." [10]

Anne Sexton's developmental experience is complicated by almost certainly having been sexually abused by her alcoholic father, perhaps from as early as age five or six. He was verbally abusive when drunk, spanked her and seems also to have been sexually intrusive, as Anne's dissociated "Elizabeth" persona wanted to testify in therapy. Elizabeth was the "little bitch" of her father's creation when he fondled her sexually. Anne was more gently abused by a cuddling caretaker aunt "Nana" to whom she turned for solace amidst family confusions.[11] Sexual overstimulation and humiliation also traced to genital inspections by her mother. "In many ways, her mother was the dangerous relationship", Dr. Orne had commented.[12] Sexton's biographer Diane Middlebrook allows only that "biochemical imbalances throughout her life intensified the underlying psychological vulnerabilities that were the primary focus of her psychotherapy".[13] Disordered biochemistry needs to be interpreted in light of the disturbed relationships especially, that with her mother, not the reverse.

Anne's hyperactive sexual imagination—what Middlebrook calls her "sexiness"—her attraction to women as well as men, should be noted. It is, in part, traceable to ambivalent attachment to her mother, who was both overstimulating and dismissive. Ambitious for Anne, she was also envious of her talent and became a rival poet. Competition and envy are precursors of manic depression, according to Cohen and Gibson. Anne identified with her mother as "solid", yet had deeper, more ambiguous feelings about her. She wrote: "I think my father was kind of crazy, though not overtly. If you tapped my father he fell apart like a jigsaw puzzle. But my mother was solid and that's what I want to be".[14] The solidity was deceptive; Anne's mother's reactions could change disconcertingly. As Anne's sister Jane is reported as saying, "you never knew, with mother, when she was going to be horrible or nice. The minute you thought you knew where you were, she'd turn on you.[15] In a sense Anne was 'twinned' with her mother against her drunken, nasty father; but she was also anxiously attached due to her mother's switch from affection to "coldness and indifference".[16] The puzzled, hurt feelings about maternal attachment come out in such poems as "Hurry Up Please It's Time" in the line "Cradle, you are a grave place"[17] As an adult Anne wrote:

"Mother makes me sick but I love her", the plight of someone unable to trust but biologically programmed to need trust.[18]

Anne Sexton was too seriously damaged to recover sufficiently from manic-depressive disorder and to move on to successful marriage and parenting; she seems not to have come to terms with bisexual urges.[19] Similarly her hopes for poetry were greater than could be realized: "Poetry led me by the hand out of madness. I am hoping I can show others that route".[20] The phrase "led me by the hand" is touchingly child-like, but there had been nobody in her childhood she could fully trust, and even the graphic psychological realism of her best poetry could not supply the secure base for relationships that had never been built.

Like Anne Sexton, Sylvia Plath had been too seriously damaged in childhood for poetry, or even poetry in conjunction with therapy, to save her from self-subverting choices in life. While there is no evidence of sexual abuse, at age eight, Plath was emotionally disabled by the death of her father and by mismanagement of what should have been healthy mourning. Throughout her life, Plath suffered the emotional parasitism of her well-meaning mother. There is no doubt that Aurelia Schober Plath did her best for her two children after the unexpected death of her husband Otto. She not only parented, but had to support the family as Otto Plath, a Boston University professor of entomology, was insufficiently insured. As Otto Plath had not sought medical help for diabetes that might have been managed, his daughter came to think of him as a sort of suicide. Many years younger than her husband, Aurelia Plath put her energies into teaching and parenting, but the emotional toll on her daughter was devastating. As first generation Americans, isolated because of wartime dislike of Germans, yet imbued with Horatio Alger aspirations to success, the Plaths meet the first Cohen-Gibson criterion for psychogenesis of bipolar disorder. There is no doubt that the acknowledged prodigy Sylvia was delegated to strive for the academic success which would lead the family out of poverty and obscurity. By an early age Sylvia had internalized a fiercely driven competitiveness, engaging in envious rivalry with other students and aspiring writers.

Sylvia craved a continuous "success story" that could be reported to her mother in the most fulsome terms, as evidenced in *Letters Home* (1975). She needed a "competitive edge", but it was another edge that troubled her —the feared disintegration that went with dangerously troubled relations with men. Her marriage with the poet Ted Hughes failed in part because of confused negative feelings about her father, so complicated and crushing to her self- esteem was her driven sexuality and marital unhappiness that suicide seemed deliverance. The brilliant poem "Edge", one of her last if not the last of her life, conveys the desperation of Plath's relational plight, chronic anxiety and fear in all relationships. It belongs to a series in the *Ariel* collection that develop a mythology of anxious inner states, so extreme that death seems the only resolution. There is little in her production to call healthy, unless a few poems concerning her children such as "Balloons".

As Plath's fate became a key issue for feminists, accurate understanding has been confounded by ideology. Also the "mad genius" identity has been thrust upon her by those wishing immunity from the emotional wreckage of her life. They point to evidence from her novel *The Bell Jar* of girlhood suicidal breakdown and hospitalization, along with such poems as "Lady Lazarus" to illustrate a sinister triumphalism of suicidal thinking right through her life. The Sylvia Plath who seemed such a brilliant success was indeed severely disturbed and too complicated a challenge for the therapies of her time. Even excellent therapists, such as Dr. Ruth Beuscher, could not lead her beyond hatred and resentment of her mother and the guilt which hate engendered. Therapy brought such feelings into awareness: "Mother's clutch. I mask my self-abasement (a transferred hate of her) and weave it with my own real dissatisfactions".[21] Her therapy seems not to have gone much beyond this, and she again needed her mother as her marriage to Ted Hughes disintegrated.

Plath's underlying psychological organization was undoubtedly bipolar, with a strong depressive component from unmourned grief for her father. The most psychologically productive of her poems, such as "Electra on the Azalea Path", openly work with grief and guilt. Plath's depression has thus long been recognized, while the bipolarity has been largely unrecognized. Bipolarity is more than merely an artifact of the wish by some to relegate Plath's indictments of certain persons by pathologizing her psyche. Like the rages her father had in his illness, Plath's poetry is sometimes rageful, and outbursts of violent hostility are recorded by a biographer.[22] Plath wrote of her bipolarity: "It is as if my life were magically run by two electric currents: joyous positive and despairing negative—which ever is running at the moment dominates my life, floods it".[23] At the end of Plath's life, separated and isolated with her children in a cold London flat, those who knew her remarked on "swift changes of mood", as if rapid cycling were setting in. If so, the risk of impulsive suicide was much increased, but Plath had not yet been able to resume the therapy which was her hope. As Sexton said of herself, poetry was a life-line; for Plath poetry was a religious calling. She wrote of it as "a religious act . . . an ordering, a reforming, a relearning and reloving of people and the world as they are and as they might be"—but maladaptive patterns were too ingrained for realization of her ideal, and poetry itself became obsessive death-circuit thinking, to use David Holbrook's phrase. [24]

The deaths of poets by suicide seem to negate any reparative or regenerative function their art might have had. Yet the impulse was healthy to express suffering rather than endure it in mute silence. The communication gap was addressed by confessional poetry, even if the art of despair made a death circuit rather than tap into reserves of healthy attachment. The poetry of Lowell, Sexton and Plath leads us to rethink depression, especially the bipolar variety, in the light of developmental experiences. The Cohen-Gibson psychogenic model is capable of reconsideration and modification in the light of recent attachment research on mother-child interactions. These research findings clarify the meanings of sensitivity, vulnerability and provoking factors in depressions, to which series "creativity" now needs to be added. Genetic predisposition and neurochemical changes would then assume a more modest place in theory of depression and its treatment. Studies such as Nancy Andreasen's and Kay Jamison's, which so severely compromise creativity as a means of discovering emotions originating in interpersonal developmental failures, would give way to improved psychobiography. Wide-angle psychiatric diagnostic exercises such as Felix Post's are important. The myth of "genius", and certainly of "mad genius", needs reappraisal.

The biographies consulted on the tragic lives of poets Lowell, Sexton and Plath could be enriched were they to use attachment theory. It could be shown that early death by suicide was the outcome of compounded developmental failures reaching back to the earliest anxious attachment to mothers, fathers and others in the milieus. Mutually illuminating comments on the creative urge and anxious attachments, including losses, would have been possible even at this comparatively early stage in the elaboration of attachment theory. Certainly the angry, obsessive defences against depression could be illuminated were the premises of attachment theory accepted. Once labelled "speculative", studies of parental loss and suicide and, more recently, of sexual abuse and suicide, can no longer be discounted. For the pioneer attachment theorist, John Bowlby, liability to childhood and adult depression is greatly increased by separations in early mother-infant interaction, and critically so by mother loss. As Bowlby wrote, "loss of mother before the tenth or eleventh birthday, when combined with certain other conditions, can play a causal role in the development of depressive disorder".[25] By "certain other conditions" Bowlby meant failures of grieving and mourning for the lost mother; in other words, failure by caregivers to encourage the natural reparative and integrative processes that give meaning to loss, can set up later depression for the child. But Bowlby had little to say about early traumatic loss of father, or about the possible consequent skewing of maternal relationship to children. Nor did he talk about the results of maternal denigration of living fathers, a probable factor among others in the psychogenesis of bipolar disorder.

Supplementing Bowlby's contribution, Jeremy Holmes points out that while early loss strongly predisposes toward later depression, the majority of depressives come from intact families. He cites a study by G. Parker on "Parental 'Affectionless' Control" (1983) as an antecedent to adult depression, that is, low care combined with overprotection, by which the intact family produces neurotic depression in certain offspring. Holmes points out that affectionless control erodes the secure base needed by a developing child, at the same time as inhibiting the free exploration necessary for a sense of competence and self-esteem.[26] This is another developmental scenario in which maternal over-control may be observed, as it is in the Cohen-Gibson theory of manic-depression's relationship with ambitious drivenness. Holmes thus shifts emphasis from outright loss to varieties of manipulation which deny the child authentic selfhood. He writes: "People with borderline personality disorder and depressive disorders regularly report the constellation of low care and high intrusiveness ('affectionless control')".[27] Thus appears a need for elaboration of Bowlby's original attachment categories for anxious attachment to include intrusive mothering styles. The work of Mary Main and Patricia Crittenden in particular shows the way forward for psychobiographies as complicated as those involving creativity in sometimes tragic lives. A more realistic appraisal is needed of poets such as Lowell,

Sexton and Plath—somewhere between outmoded "artist hero" and inconsequential "sick poet". Each had the courage to reveal childhood traumas in loss and abuse and to enact a self-healing plan through poetic creativity. They sought symbolic means to self-regulate and contain in words massive anxiety with discernable origin in actual experience. Obsessively willful and narcissistic though their self-presentations may often be, healthy impulses are also discerned when profiles of attachment experience are considered.

Guidance in formulating believable psychobiography is found in such papers as Murray Parkes's "Separation Anxiety: An Aspect of the Search for a Lost Object" and such books as Vamik D. Volkan's *Linking Objects and Linking Phenomena.*[28] These studies help to discern symbolic representations of anxiety themes in art and to connect them to life events throughout development. More broadly, loss of attachments to parents needs to be seen in the psycho-social perspective supplied by George W. Brown, Tirril Harris and John R. Copeland in "Depression and Loss" (1977) and subsequent writings.[29] These studies look at depression not as mysterious biochemical disorganization but as emotional states directly connected to adverse life circumstances from earliest "sensitivity" factors, through "vulnerability" to "provoking" agents. The studies urge that life-review is necessary to understand any instance of depression, but especially those of the unipolar type. While Brown and Harris did not study bipolar disorder, their general principles apply, and careful research strategies such as theirs are needed to carry forward promising "hunches" gained from the work of Cohen and Gibson. Finally, George Engel's "conservation-withdrawal" theory of depression as a means of incubating solutions to seemingly insoluble problems of relationship should be considered in connection with the arts. Each poem or picture on an anxious theme may be seen as a sort of proto-depressed withdrawal to reorganize disorganized attachments to persons, places and events.[30] Incorporation of negative, anxiety-causing experiences into a framework of new meaning is the task of creativity, and accurate psychobiography makes it understandable.

Notes

1. Ian Hamilton, *Robert Lowell: A Biography* (New York: Vintage, 1983), p. 473.

2. Ian Hamilton, "The Embarrassing Pursuit," *Times Literary Supplement*, April 29, 1994, p. 17.

3. Ian Hamilton, *Robert Lowell: A Biography*, p. 216.

4. Ibid., p. 404.

5. Ibid., p. 5.

6. Ibid., p. 13.

7. Ibid., p. 9.

8. Ibid., pp. 28–9. The nickname Cal was part Caligula, part Caliban, suggesting the coarser side of Lowell's nature (see ibid., pp. 19–20).

9. Diane Middlebrook, *Anne Sexton: A Biography* (Boston: Houghton Mifflin, 1991), p. 61; *Anne Sexton: A Self-Portrait in Letters*, ed., Linda Sexton and Lois Ames (Boston: Houghton Mifflin, 1977), p. 40.

10. Ibid., p. 224.

11. Ibid., p. 56f. Joshua Kendall and Alan Plotkin point out how ineffective Anne Sexton's psychotherapy actually was because it failed to take into account early sexual abuse (*Treating Abuse Today*, 5, no. 2 (1995): 27). For discussion of failure to diagnose Sexton's Dissociative Identity Disorder see Colin A. Ross, M.D., *The Osiris complex: Case-Studies in Multiple Personality Disorder* (Toronto: University of Toronto Press, 1994). Not only were Sexton's therapists unequipped to help her much, so was the literary world blind to the implications of her poetry. Ross writes, "the poetry is morbid, unhealthy and extremely limited in range, rhythm, emotional depth and energy. Anne Sexton's work is the poetry of a single alter personality and of an organism heading to suicide: it taps only a tiny subregion of the whole human

being's memory, experience, thought and feeling. The world might be more enriched if it had a volume of Elizabeth's writing to read", Elizabeth being Sexton's child "alter" personality who held memories of paternal incest (p. 212).

12. Ibid., p. 59.

13. Ibid., p. 37.

14. Ibid., p. 49.

15. Ibid., p. 13.

16. Ibid., p. 38.

17. Anne Sexton, *The Death Notebooks* (Boston: Houghton Mifflin, 1974), p. 68.

18. Middlebrook, *Anne Sexton: A Biography*, pp. 46–47.

19. For Anne Sexton's acceptance of bisexuality, see Marjorie Garber, *Vice Versa: Bisexuality and Eroticism in Everyday Life* (New York: Simon & Schuster, 1995), p. 118.

20. Anne Sexton, *A Self-Portrait in Letters*, p. 301.

21. Anne Stevenson, *Bitter Flame: A Life of Sylvia Plath* (New York: Viking, 1989), p. 147.

22. Ibid., pp. 97, 135, 193.

23. Ibid., p. 134. See also p. 280.

24. Sylvia Plath, *The Journals*, ed. Ted Hughes (New York: Dial Press, 1982), p. 272. Plath was strongly motivated to break her suicidal pattern as fictionalized in *The Bell Jar* (1963): "I must be my own doctor. I must cure this destructive paralysis and ruinous brooding and daydreaming", she wrote in her journal (p. 246). It is clear that psychotherapy with Dr. Ruth Beuscher had a freeing effect: "it makes me feel good as hell to express my hostility for my mother, frees me from the Panic Bird on my heart and my typewriter . . ." (p. 266).

Psychotherapy improved access to the sources of anxiety displayed in her poetry, but it did not actually free her of them. See David Holbrook, *Sylvia Plath: Poetry and Existence* (London: Athlone, 1976).

25. John Bowlby, *Attachment and Loss* (London: Hogarth, 1980), vol. 3, *Loss, Sadness and Depression*, p. 215. For recent critical refinements of Bowlby's study see Kenneth S. Adam et al., "Vulnerability to Loss, Separation and Abuse" in *Attachment Theory: Social, Developmental, and Clinical Perspectives*, ed. S. Goldberg et al. (Hillsdale, N. J., The Analytic Press, 1995) p. 329f.

26. Jeremy Holmes, *John Bowlby and Attachment Theory* (London: Routledge, 1993), p. 187.

27. Ibid., p. 223.

28. C. Murray Parkes, "Separation Anxiety: An Aspect of the Search for a Lost Object," *Studies in Anxiety*, ed. by M. H. Leder (London: Headley, 1969); Vamik D. Volkan, *Linking Objects and Linking Phenomena* (New York: International Universities Press, 1981).

29. See George W. Brown and Tirril Harris, *Social Origins of Depression* (New York: The Free Press, 1978) and subsequent confirming studies.

30. G. L. Engel and A. H. Schmale, "Conservation-Withdrawal: A Primary Regulatory Process for Organic Homeostasis," in *Physiology, Emotion and Psychosomatic Illness*, ed. R. Porter and J. Knight (Amsterdam: Elsevier-Excerpta, 1972); Engel and Schmale, "The Role of Conservation-Withdrawal in Depressive Reactions," in *Depression and Human Existence*, ed E. J. Anthony and T. Benedek (Boston: Little, Brown, 1975).

Conclusion

Attachment, Trauma and a New View of Creativity

> Beauty alone is a sovereign remedy against
> fear, grief and all melancholy fits . . .
> —Robert Burton (1621/51)

> Beauty is nothing but the beginning of terror
> that we can just barely endure, and we admire
> it so because it calmly disdains to destroy us.
> —Rainer Maria Rilke (1912/22)[1]

We would like to believe with Burton that the creation of beauty remedies fear and grief, but to say palliates, or compensates for, fear and grief would be more accurate. Hyperbolic though Rilke's twentieth century statement may sound, it corrects, if not supplants, Burton's. Creativity often reaches but seldom, if ever, permanently alleviates the core anxieties of those who create or sense beauty. Developmental and relational anxieties—even terrors—are prime motivators to creativity; they are richly encoded in created objects, whether of the plastic arts, literature or music. Aesthetic objects may be called "anxiety organizers and containers". They mimic secure attachment relations while safely enclosing in imagery cues to respond anxiously. Aesthetic objects reproduce anxiety situations in a "safe space", inviting a relaxation response to stressors. Yet aesthetic objects do not dispose of psychotoxic anxieties or necessarily improve interpersonal functions in which anxieties arise. Aesthetic experience returns us to reassuringly primitive, pre-traumatic, states reminiscent of being safely at the breast. Further, aesthetic experience temporarily resets expectations about how good attachments might be reinstated, containing anxiety provoking bad attachments in image and narrative. It is a promise of better possibilities, of better life to come, but creativity and aesthetic experience alone cannot heal; they can only reveal what needs to be healed and improve aspiration by showing an ideal paradigm of formal harmonies.

Nonetheless, artistic creativity is a defining characteristic of humankind and essential to understand if we are to make best use of what the arts have to offer. Creativity is enormously valuable as an indicator of the main anxiety situations in any era. Thematic anxieties showing in the arts indicate where the human wish for wholeness is being cramped, warped or dangerously depersonalized. The arts are often indicators of social pathology and also of wishes for healing; but artists themselves too easily become sacrificial victims. Artists generally do not like to think of creativity as confessional or as therapeutic for themselves or anyone else. They insist that the arts should be free to move in any direction, however anarchic, not constrained by requirements for anybody's moral improvement. Artists are not noted for their powers of self-preservation, despite self-preservation being the origin of creativity.

Even creative persons who affirm confessional and therapeutic intentions are likely to fall into sacrificial roles. One of this century's masters of poetic lyricism, Rilke, suffered from chronic depression and the effects of Don Juanism. He deliberately missed an opportunity for treatment by Freud (although briefly accepting that of a lesser analyst), in the belief that such masterworks as *The Duino Elegies* would heal anxieties about women and fears of death. Who knows how much worse Rilke's suffering would have been without his poetic craft, yet depression dogged him and he never found its source. Similarly the novelist Graham Greene, who reports in his autobiography a reparative analysis as a schoolboy, later realized that he suffered from manic-depressive disorder, including periods of unendurable boredom, lassitude and suicidal ideation, which no therapy of the time could reach. Greene thought of literary creativity as escape from the madness, panic fear and melancholia of the human situation, but none of his writings disclosed the source, let alone healed, the dangerous anxieties with which Greene lived his entire life. Should such examples do more than reinforce pessimism about the intractable suffering of many celebrated, but psychologically martyred, persons dedicated to lives of creativity? I do not think that we have yet thought enough about the creative urge; by doing so within the new framework of attachment theory a better set of possibilities will appear.

Evidence for strong innate repair urges from infancy onward prompt reconsideration of the problem of creativity and the importance of its products as they accumulate to define a "culture". A culture offers its members, when threatened, psychological sustainment through providing repair codes that reinstate a larger sense of meaning to which all tacitly subscribe. The arts, traditionally allied to religion, have helped to overcome doubts about the value of living, matching good internalized images with their external referents in nature, society and transcendent belief systems, while "holding" persecutory anxieties in safe aesthetic form. At least so it was in the great eras of western art from the Middle Ages throughout the Renaissance and into the nineteenth century. With the twentieth century's breakdown of the Christian-Humanist synthesis through industrialization, revolution and war, the arts weakened, and sometimes lost, their reparative function of reintegrating psychological distress into a system of shared beliefs. Surrealism, generated by total war and social upheaval in Europe, seems swamped by its sudden access of unconscious anxiety and fear. Surrealism's overwhelming sexual content suggests that its artists contacted massive upwellings of male-female relational anxieties not before dealt with in the arts. It is hard to find cultural repair codes at work in the writings of André Breton or the paintings of Max Ernst or the "sculpture" of Hans Bellmer, where anxious attachments predominate.[2]

I propose that the biological repair function of creativity be reinstated in the arts. For best effect it should be combined with meditation practice and psychotherapy, especially using guided imagery. There is a tremendous human resource in creativity being trivialized by contemporary deconstructive cynicism and commercially-driven style consciousness. If Rembrandt's seventeenth century self-portraits, or John Donne's erotic and religious lyrics, are taken as standards of authenticity, by contrast most of today's self-aware art appears inadequate. Yet the unconscious—or dissociated—sources of creativity in developmental trauma, anxious attachments and interpersonal unease are just as urgent now as then, and the means of reaching them are more exacting. Spontaneous imagery can be used psychotherapeutically to decipher core anxieties.

It is unlikely that we will return to a Christianity such as upheld Rembrandt and Donne, yet there may be a supplementary (or alternative) standard of wholeness implicit in the living organism itself. The self-repairing, self-organizing, or autopoetic, nature of living organisms, beginning at the molecular level, needs reconsideration. We should look again at the creative urge, in full developmental perspective, this time grasping what is so special about it. The creative urge belongs in a sequence with the earliest interactive means by which proximity to a caregiver is maintained. It is a displaced version of the urge for reunion with a safe caregiver, with the nurturing breast and holding by an unconditionally accepting mother. By resorting to idealized states, creativity circumvents the imperfections of actual mothering, but it preserves, and sometimes enhances, connections with inner reality. The idealized created object is homologous with the intact, harmoniously functioning human organism, the person as he or she might be at their best: *mens sana in corpore sano*. Inner reality is made more tolerable and more workable when brought as imagery into psychotherapy.

Thus concessions to the creative arts as being inter-textual, merely self-referential, belonging to a "world apart", are not helpful; quite the opposite —the arts are the best possible routes to discovering anxieties, generated by sub-optimal attachments, which perturb individuals and inhibit the growth of awareness of self in relation to others. Human destructiveness, including self-destructiveness, is now on such a scale that its developmental origins must be faced. As these origins are generally hidden from ourselves, a major route of access is by fantasies produced by artists, including group fantasy. Each of the arts, including film, yields anxious fantasies, arising from dissociated affect, which common sense viewing is likely to miss. Before looking at some examples of what psychobiographical criticism reveals of creative attempts to penetrate sources of anxiety, let us briefly review what psychobiology understands of reparative processes.

Attachment-like behaviors are observable in mammals well before actual attachment comes into operation. Myron Hofer gives experimental evidence that "mutual regulation, synchrony, and reciprocity are built into mammalian mother-infant interactions at a deep biological level".[3] Hofer uses "state organization, symbiosis, and the biphasic approach-withdrawal theory" to show how affect arises in infant-mother interaction.[4] He describes how regulatory interactions "appear to be capable of inducing the searching and proximity-seeking behavior directed toward an increasingly specific object that is the hallmark of attachment behavior".[5] Hofer comments that "Regulation is apparent at all levels of biological organization within individuals, ranging from molecules to organ systems", from which it follows that relationally governed homeostatic controls are essential to maintaining life.[6] The acute anxiety caused by infant separation from mother described by Bowlby is thus grounded by Hofer in still earlier behaviors established through evolution. Proximity-seeking behaviors confer fitness for survival on the young of every species. Here we recall Thomas Hunt Morgan's basic work on tissue repair and how every organism is programmed to restore lost or impaired function. At the level of attachment the same principle holds, but outcomes are far more risky. What happens when proximity to the caregiver conveys weak, unclear or outright distressing messages—when neuroanatomy is either understimulated, overloaded or confused? In humans, the lasting neuroanatomical and behavioral effects of insecure attachments in infancy are being clarified, the basic research having been reviewed in earlier chapters. Less appreciated, but central to understanding creativity, are the repair mechanisms observable in a hierarchy of complexity and sophistication. To start with the simplest, stressful reunion behavior, when an infant fusses and cries may prompt mother to soothe and comfort, modifying her earlier perceived rejectiveness. Attachment is restored reparatively; that is, a lastingly useful means of easing distress may have been discovered. This interactive repair may become a repeatable means of restoring secure attachment, or perhaps not, in which case more elaborate—defensively designed— intrapsychic, or subjective, techniques will arise in the infant. Now anxiety has been internalized, making repair more problematic. Nonetheless an innate urge to repair and restore secure attachment will be enhanced, effortful and frustrating though it proves to be. Both the mother and infant try harder, either reducing or escalating tension. As Allan N. Schore writes, these adaptations are pre-verbal, encoding directly into the infant's neuroarchitecture. Schore's technical summary is: "that practicing phase-specific, external, interpersonal, caregiver-modulated arousal regulation, especially after stress-induced dyadic mismatches (attachment breaks), specifically influences the experience dependent maturation of orbitofrontal structure which underlies and supports internal, intrapersonal regulatory functions subserved by prefrontal internal working models".[7] The sobering point here is that the infant's early maladaptive experience becomes neurologically encoded in ways that are very difficult to modify. Every organic system has the capability of self-regulation and renewal; eyes blink, the stomach digests its contents, cuts heal and sleep restores energy; but psychological adaptations are learned patterns of response, initiated by mothers who teach their infants "how to feel". If the feelings are dysphoric, arduous special techniques are needed to modify them: hence the invention of psychotherapy and the endless debate as to how to make it most effective.

For Schore, shame reactions—the infant's self-blame for failed attachments—are the primary source of psychopathology. This suggests that shame variants should be looked for in each of anxious avoidant, ambivalent and disorganized deviations from secure attachment. Schore shows that the quality of mother-infant eye contact is growth-promoting or inhibiting. He writes that "the autoregulation of shame may depend on the internalization of the 'mirroring' positive affect amplifying function of the maternal gleam".[8] Such preverbal feeling states, conveyed by looking and seeing, are not easily recovered into awareness. The unconscious lacks a formal language, necessitating the creative invention of feeling-toned visual and verbal images to approximate and to represent such experiences. Expressing these primitive feeling-toned images in the language of art, music or literature is a later, very sophisticated, achievement. The artist's search for self-transcendence and higher consciousness in imagery and language is often traceable this far back in development, although the biographical pathway from traumatized attachment to aesthetic achievement needs interpretation by a sound theory of development.

Psychobiographically understood, artistic creativity is a late emerging means of assisting with affect regulation, the management of developmental sensitivities to environmental stressors which threaten to dysregulate emotions. Creativity produces mental representations, in image and word, of states of anxiety and tension needing regulation. By objectifying anxiety in mental representations—which can be transferred onto canvas or printed page—creativity controls the extremes of affect: depression or mania. But self-initiated mood control is no simple matter as we now know that brain structures are involved which do not easily yield to internal or external influences. Indeed, their very defensive design is to resist influences and, the more rigid defences are, the more "stuck", the less chance there is for self-initiated modification and the more resistance to psychotherapy. Hence, instead of productive self-repair, the artist may narcissistically compensate for suffering, which remains unmodified, or even compounds itself through repetition and amplification of imaging. As has been remarked, fortunate is the artist operating in the A/C defensive mode, combining avoidance with controlling ambivalence, as he or she has a measure of adaptive flexibility. It is, however, unknown just what proportion of creative persons actually have A/C personality organization—a matter for further study. In severe disruption of attachment, as when mother dies and the infant must adapt to alternative caretakers, relational repair becomes suddenly complicated. Loss of "contact comfort" and of the very source of facial recognition and affirmative "eye gleam" is a critical test for reparative resources. Early loss of father, throwing the infant or child exclusively into mother's care, has a different but equally fateful set of developmental consequence for both boys and girls. Loss of both parents has yet further relational complications in substitute parenting. The experimental studies of Marvin Eisenstadt et al. on parental loss and achievement show that the traumas of early parental loss can stimulate later high achievement in the arts, sciences, and statesmanship. My own studies of mother-dominated sons in *Obsession and Culture: A Study of Sexual Obsession in Modern Fiction* assess the reparative distortions in the fantasies of Jocasta-reared sons who become creative writers. Consistent through all these scenarios of loss and replacement of attachment figures is the infant or child's urgent, but too often thwarted, wish to make good the deficit. [9]

Many instances spring to mind of art manifesting obvious anxiety, as if pleading with viewer or reader for empathic engagement with its troubled presence. Some examples follow in which beginnings have been made in the discovery of the experiential background of creativity. For instance, the Norwegian expressionist Edvard Munch's (1863–1944) self-portraits, from *Self-Portrait with a Cigarette* (1895) to self-portraits of the 1940s are intensely anxious and melancholic. Munch's *The Cry* (1893) is perhaps the most famous image of desperation in the modern world. What lay behind his distress, and why was it never alleviated, although, as he said, he hoped that his art would bring him "a light out of darkness"? Carol M. Ravenal writes of Munch's "need to find grace through forming aesthetic wholes out of his traumata, . . . initially triggered by the conflicted and split feelings surrounding the early death of his mother when he was five".[10] Ravenal's psychobiographical reconstruction of Munch's entire family constellation convincingly shows sources of his depressive sense of maternal loss, of later debilitating overstimulation, and explains why and how Munch used painting to strive for "a more cohesive self-image". Mary Mathews Gedo's *Picasso: Art as Autobiography* (1980) similarly examines Picasso's early life for evidence of trauma since Picasso's anxiety about women and sexuality pervades his paintings over many decades. A superstar of modern art, Picasso (1881–1973) was as notorious for his many marriages and sexual relationships as he was famous for revolutionizing painting in the twentieth century. Gedo examines Picasso's relations with his not very successful artist father and with his "tenacious" and "tyrannical" mother whom he had to escape by leaving Spain. Picasso's attraction to beautiful but vulnerable women prompts Gedo to speculate about relations with his mother. She finds his self-esteem unusually vulnerable, suggesting that Picasso had the sort of mother "particularly prone to aggrandize their young male children, and to involve them in a kind of symbiotic enmeshment from which the child cannot extricate himself... This constellation occurs all the more readily if a young mother is married to a man many years her senior, as was the case with Picasso's parents".[11] Picasso's obsessively extreme ambivalence about women as either "goddesses" or "doormats" played out through many tormented relationships imaged in his paintings, including those of "monster women" in which huge, grotesque forms are made sexually repulsive. Gedo studies both Picasso's female and male affiliations in the light of his narrow escape from domination by his mother. She makes life-art connection intelligible and convincingly accounts for the high levels of anxiety in both.

Picasso's aggressive distortions of the female form, as in *Nude in an Armchair* (1929) or *Woman Dressing her Hair* (1940) find their male analogue in the homoerotic paintings of Francis Bacon (1909-1992). The obsessive intensity and daring of Bacon's distortions of both male and female forms are even greater than Picasso's, and the anguish is unrelieved by such sexually playful moments as are sometimes found in Picasso's paintings. For example, Bacon's smeared and contorted portraits of his lover George Dyer, who committed suicide, achieve a sort of ruined dignity; the paintings' brilliant spontaneity of execution reinforces their relational nihilism, and sadomasochistic violence is ever present. Reconstructions of Bacon's

Anglo-Irish childhood have begun. As a reviewer wrote, Bacon's biographer, Andrew Sinclair attempts "to trace the origin of this obsession with violence", discovering childhood experiences, including "Bacon's father having Francis horse-whipped by his grooms and finding his son dressed in his wife's underclothes". Sinclair also tried to discover Bacon's complicated relations with his nanny, whose death left him inconsolable.[12] By such psychobiographical contextualizing, Bacon's obsessive annihilations of human faces and forms begin to make sense.

The writer Franz Kafka (1883–1924) is probably the most effective chronicler of anxiety in western literature. Kafka's stories, such as "The Metamorphosis" and his "Letter to His Father" (1919) perform an autoanalysis of an oppressed childhood that had left Kafka in emotional turmoil and unable to marry. In "The Metamorphosis" the child Gregor Samsa is transformed into a lowly cockroach and views his persecutory family from that perspective, whereas in the "Letter" Kafka speaks in his own voice protesting his abusive father and cringing mother, although his sisters were relatively more benign. Kafka was a middle European Jew who shared the same ethos that produced psychoanalysis. He was also a mythopoeic genius who epitomized modern anxiety; in *The Castle* and *The Trial* bafflement as to the meaning of existence prevails. Kafka knew that anxiety and feelings of the absurdity of life had relational origins, although he was unable completely to discover the origin of his thematic obsessions. Studies such as Margarete Mitscherlich-Nielsen's "Psychoanalytic Notes on Franz Kafka, the Psychobiography of a Disturbed Genius" assist in making sense of the more conventional biographies, the sociocultural and family reconstruction by Ronald Hayman, for example.[13]

Of all celebrated modern writing, perhaps attitudes to the work of novelist Ernest Hemingway (1899–1961) have been most affected by biographical and psychobiographical studies. Hemingway's once-accepted self-presentation as America's most virile writer is now seen as exhibiting a deep anxiety about sexual orientation. Kenneth S. Lynn's *Hemingway* (1987) brought to view disturbing features of childhood development that helped explain Hemingway's sexual preoccupations in his life and fiction. A bizarre obsessively bi-sexual short hair fetish had come to light the previous year with publication of Hemingway's reconstructed manuscript

The Garden of Eden, and bisexual preoccupation was detected elsewhere in his fiction. In Lynn's view, "Uncertain to the point of fear about himself, [Hemingway] was compelled to write stories in which he endeavored to cope with the disorder of his inner world by creating fictional equivalents for it".[14] As Hemingway could not make secure adult attachments (he had four wives), suffered from depression and died by suicide, Lynn and other biographers have felt justified in tracing his anxiety about life to the earliest anxious attachments to parents in the family setting. Although not an analyst, Lynn promisingly hypothesizes about Hemingway being effeminized by his domineering mother—who dressed him as a girl to twin with a sister—and being distressed by a bipolar father who eventually took his own life. It turns out that hyper-masculine Hemingway, who was always trying to prove himself by feats of courage and daring, was anxiously bisexual, using fiction to try to resolve his relational dilemma. [15]

Hemingway detested psychoanalysis, but Samuel Beckett (1906–1989), arguably the most important post-Second–World–War European playwright, was released by analytic treatment to do his best work. Beckett is remembered as the most original of all artists who evoked existential anxiety—anxiety about 'being' itself. His biographer, Deirdre Bair, revealed that during 1934–1935 Beckett was in analysis in London with Wilfred R. Bion, a revisionist Kleinian whose theories of language as communication strongly influenced him.[16] In fact Beckett and Bion were mutually influential to the enrichment of both art and psychodynamic theory. Readings of Beckett's *Waiting for Godot* (1955) and *Endgame* (1958) profit by knowledge of schizoid split-egos and Bion's understanding of how language functions in emotional disturbance. The extent of Beckett's anxious relations with his Dublin parents, especially his mother, can be gauged from the psychoanalytic commentary on these despairing yet brilliantly comic plays. The extent of Beckett's autobiographical, self-analytic preoccupation is being realized in commentaries not only on the nihilistic novels but especially on such probing treatments of family relations as *Eleutheria, A Dream of Fair to Middling Women* and *Company*.

All-in all, the foregoing examples from painting and literature show how urgently needed is a theory of creativity as attempted redirection from the artist's sub-optimal developmental pathways. When the artist's biography is taken into account, the problems of anxiety in relationships begin to come into focus; clues gather as to his or her fantasy, dominant themes and "obsessive metaphors", as the critic Charles Mauron called them.[17] The critic's work is thus redirected toward the actual developmental and subsequent attachments which have motivating force in creativity.

Two questions arise: first, how can it be said that creativity in the arts is always an emergency response to anxiety when evidence is lacking for such an assertion? Where is anxiety in the tranquil seventeenth century Dutch domestic interior painting of Pieter de Hooch or Johannes Vermeer? Where is anxiety in Henry Fielding's high-spirited eighteenth century masterpiece *Tom Jones*, or in Alexander Pope's brilliant mock-epic *The Rape of the Lock*? Apart from standard plot and character conflicts, much literature cannot be said to exhibit anything like anxiety; nor is anxiety easily detected in the western tradition of domestic and landscape painting. Yet when there seems to be no overt anxiety the rule should be to "look deeper". Pieter de Hooch died in the Amsterdam insane asylum and Vermeer, who had fifteen children of his own, is not known ever to have painted a child. Henry Fielding is among many writers who lost a mother early, at age eleven; he made his fictional hero Tom Jones a foundling. Alexander Pope's poetic asperity is that of a congenitally deformed person who easily felt himself mocked. In much literature anxiety is very evident. For instance, it pervades the erotic and religious verse of John Donne, while in the aftermath of the English revolution John Milton wrote an epic, *Paradise Lost*, in which he anxiously reviewed the Christian promise of redemption to fallen man.

There are sometimes dangerous highwaymen in Claude Lorraine's Virgilian landscape visions, and menace of one sort or another can be expected throughout the works of European Romanticism. But as long as Christian-Humanism gave reassurances of larger metaphysical containment of the evil in human affairs, anxiety did not threaten to overwhelm subject matter in the arts. It is in the post-Christian-Humanist early modern and modern eras of increasingly individualistic aloneness that anxiety becomes a dominant theme—sometimes more than the arts can contain as in German Expressionist painting. The unspeakable horror of the Holocaust and the devising and use of thermonuclear weapons seems to exceed containment by reparative creativity. Further, in an era of anonymity and alienation, it is often difficult reliably to reconstruct motivations to creativity when early life data is controversial or not obtainable. For this reason alone, the hypothesis that all art is a self-healing adaptive response to dangerously stressed attachments is risky. It is offered as a project to be studied, given the limitations of data and the realization that theory of adult attachment behavior is still being developed. This study asserts that questions of attachment-motivated creativity are answerable for many artists and that larger patterns of causality are established.

The second question is whether in the light of so much suffering and self-destructiveness among creative persons, as we know from biographies, the idea of 'regeneration' or 'repair' is not, after all, irrelevant. What is the point of mentioning an innate urge to health and wholeness if anxiety and despair finally triumph, ending life in absurdity or tragedy? Are there examples of actual reparative or regenerative transformations among artists,writers and musicians—where the result is more than temporary consolation for and accommodation to disorder, a sort of palliative self-care? Surely it is too simple to call creativity a dialysis device for purifying the emotions of toxic attachments, when we know that no final purification is possible and, as with dialysis, that in the absence of healthy structures the toxins only build up again. It may be thought that there remains little that creativity can do for accumulated anxious attachments in the artist and secondarily in the recipient of the art product. Creativity can, however, portray an "ideally ordered aesthetic space" for imaginative aspiration. It can also deliver into its maker's consciousness manageable instalments of the toxic emotions which complete the cycle of personal "story". This in turn may lead to an accommodation with depressive, self-destroying feelings, or ego weakness, in psychodynamic terminology. Dreams, introspection, meditation, symbolization in the arts—all can deliver authentic feelings about chronically distressing anxious attachments. The closer to completion and acceptance the "story" comes (most favorably with analytic assistance), the more likelihood of increments in lasting health. Lest this be branded a new Philistinism, it should be remarked that historically the arts have been part of traditional healing, more or less actively invoked in ritual cures, which scientific scepticism tends to set aside without understanding their power. There are many examples of regenerative outcomes of creativity to offset the mainly negative examples cited. The most persuasive of them are historic, especially in the English seventeenth century when Christianity was still a force. Each of the so-called metaphysical poets, John Donne (1572–1631),

George Herbert (1593–1633) and Henry Vaughan (1621–1695) had a profound spiritual and psychological upheaval and reordering, recorded in the poetry; each passed from secular ambition and amorousness to religious commitment. In the cases of Donne and Herbert penitential fidelity to devotional practice and church affiliation deepened their lives, while in Vaughan's case renunciation of his "follies" led to astonishing mystical awareness which appears in poems of nature foreshadowing Romantic pantheism. The idea of spiritual repair was still potent. Repenting Donne spoke directly to God:

> Thou hast made me, And shall thy work decay?
> Repaire me now, for now mine end doth haste,
> I runne to death, and death meets me as fast,
> And all my pleasures are like yesterday.
> (Holy sonnet, I)

George Herbert's devotional poetry proves experientially that "Fractures well cur'd make us more strong" ("Repentance"). Henry Vaughan questioned a simple flower about its annual rebirth as a figure of spiritual regeneration, learning that living underground, the flower:

> Did there repaire
> Such losses as befel him in this air
> And would e'r long
> Come forth most fair and young
> ("I walkt the other day. . .")

The model for these conversions was St. Paul, with St. Augustine's *Confessions* of sin and regeneration another memorable instance. The English seventeenth century supplies other equally impressive examples of the self-proclaimed malcontent or sinner regenerated, as in *The Journal* of George Fox or John Bunyan's *Grace Abounding to the Chief of Sinners*. In each instance religious melancholia, or depression (bipolar in Bunyan), was overcome, or at least alleviated, by the conversion experience. We would, of course, like to know more about predisposing anxious parental attachments than can now be recovered. Our difference from the seventeenth century is in lacking a securely held framework of meaning, a "symbolic order" to encourage such acts of faith. Perhaps our symbolic order is the intrinsic ordering of the cell which allows life in complex organisms; cellular developmental and regenerative powers may be mystery enough to support the argument about creativity.

It is no doubt unrealistic to look for complete and lasting cures from emotional disorder among poets, but there are examples of significant alleviations and postponements of relapse. The suicidal poet William Cowper (1731–1800) traced his melancholia to loss of his mother at age six, and to misfortunes of caretaking thereafter. His deep insight into the source of suffering appears in the elegy "On Receipt of My Mother's Picture Out of Norfolk" (1790); there is no doubt that Cowper kept himself alive by writing whimsical, diverting but sometimes deeply insightful verse. Other eighteenth century writers such as Samuel Johnson and Christopher Smart more or less successfully used literature to stave off depression. The Romantic poet William Wordsworth, whose mother died when he was eight, felt an aching loneliness which was partially assuaged by intense experiences of nature in his native Lake country. "The Prelude" (1805/revised 1850) poignantly relives experiences of boyhood among the hills, and the poem expressly develops the idea of the mind's inherent healing powers:

> The mind of man is framed even like the breath
> and harmony of music; there is a dark
> Inscrutable workmanship that reconciles
> Discordant elements, makes them cling together
> In one society.[18]

Wordsworth's anxiety and depression were certainly controlled to an extent impossible had he not continuously written poetry tracking changing states of feeling. The process of mourning can be greatly enhanced by such expressive writing and, although elegy seems out of fashion, there are enough examples, from Henry King's "An Exequy to His Matchless Never to Be Forgotten Friend", his wife, Anne, who died in 1624, to Douglas Dunn's *Elegies* (1985), following the death from cancer of his young wife, Lesley, to show a reparative function by enabling mourning. The most complex and searching example of this genre is probably Thomas Hardy's series of fifty-eight lyrics of recreated ideal love, guilt and remorse for estrangement following the death in 1912 of his wife, Emma. Each poem, or set of poems, chronicles the emotional meaning to the poet of love and loss, indeed of the attachments that activated his own deepest anxieties.

Examples from other arts could be given, for instance Gustav Mahler's use of music to come to terms with his deep anxiety about mortality arising from losses of family in his childhood. These exercises in creativity might in many instances be termed palliative self-care for trauma, or merely consolation for irrecoverable loss, but they do illustrate the point about the reparative urge to mourn extending from soma to psyche. The often sentimental memorial verses published with newspaper obituaries serve much the same healing function. Works such as Sylvia Fraser's *My Father's House* (about discovering early sexual abuse by her father) and Marie Cardinal's autobiographical novel *The Words to Say It* (about the successful psychotherapy of a woman who had been an unwanted child) are leading examples of creativity as repair. Although subject to controversy over the reliability of recovered memories, such work points towards understanding attachment as the leading feature of human biology. Psychodynamic insights into loss and mourning have led to such valuable studies as Esther Dreifuss-Kattan's *Cancer Stories: Creativity and Self-Repair* (1990). These studies of cancer patients' creative responses in painting and writing to the devastating results of surgery bring to the forefront of healing the innate creative urge to restore wholeness and wellness—even facing death. Dreifuss-Kattan extends the concept of healing much beyond its conventional medical meaning.

These reparative statements belong to the confessional genre, already alluded to. Originally a religious exercise, the confession of wrongdoing and repentance, and of conversion to a faith (beginning with St. Augustine's *Confessions* c. 400) has had a long history in the Christian church. Psychological interest in states of mind revealed in spiritual confessions, appearing as early as the seventeenth century, arises from the high incidence of depression. Concern with mood disorders in religion contributed to psychological enquiry, which in turn prepared the way for psychoanalysis. Confession is obviously linked to Freud's "talking cure", a major shaping force in modern literature.[19] Thus confession—telling in words heard by another of one's deepest and most troubling secrets—became a staple of both psychodynamic treatments and their simulation in fiction.

Unrecognized until recently, however, is the extent to which confession actually improves not only mental health but health altogether. Originally designed to give evidence of salvation replacing damnation, and of catharsis for depressive moods, confession is now seen to tone the mind-body's neurochemistry. In an impressive experimental study, "Disclosure of Traumas and Immune Function: Health Implications for Psychotherapy", James W. Pennebaker et al., showed that inhibition of stressful feeling and thought can be relieved by confession and thereby improve immune-system function. Pennebaker writes, "Individuals who are forced to confront upsetting experiences in their lives show improvements in physical health relative to control subjects. More important, in our study the individuals who showed the greatest health improvements were those who wrote about topics that they had actively held back from telling others.[20] Experts on trauma, such as Judith Herman, confirm that "the attempt to avoid reliving the trauma too often results in a narrowing of consciousness, a withdrawal from engagement with others, and an impoverished life".[21] Pennebaker has gone on to advocate "confession. as a relief from anxiety", that is, an opening up through expressive writing of the most closed and constricted experiences which generate anticipations of renewed anxious attachments.[22]

Without citing the history of confessional art and literature, Pennebaker states exactly what it shows: the search for freedom from inner persecution. Without citing research in attachment theory, he similarly shows how assumptive models of attachment (Bowlby's "working models"of interpersonal relations) can be modified for the better by writing. His simple and profound statement is: "when people confront traumas by talking or writing about them, their mental and physiological stress levels drop. Confronting traumas allows individuals to reorganize and assimilate the events".[23] Bessel van der Kolk, who studies post-traumatic stress disorder, agrees: "Once flexibility is introduced, the traumatic memory starts losing its power over current experience".[24] Of course there are methodological complications as to exactly how "expressive writing" should be conducted, and what part a therapist should play, but the principle of externalizing anxious inner states is well established.

Little wonder that expressive therapies should take a leading role in management of the controversial Dissociative Identity Disorders (DID). As the so-called "multiple personalities", usually seen in girls, are traceable to childhood sexual overstimulation, often by an interfering adult, it follows that recovering and assembling memory traces is essential to successful therapy. The pioneers in this area are Richard Kluft, MD, Frank Putnam, MD, and Colin Ross, MD, each with important theoretical statements about the techniques and efficacy of expressive therapies.[25] While the concepts of repression and dissociation are repeatedly challenged by some psychologists and psychiatrists, there is little doubt that the influences of early attachments remain largely out of awareness, and that even early traumatic insults to the attachment system may be lost as precise, easily recoverable information.

Retrieval and acknowledgment of feelings surrounding early attachments are a major achievement, as appears from the results of Mary Main's Adult Attachment Interview (AAI). Main looks for coherence of statement about child-parent interactions, testing whether all aspects of personality formation are available for expression in words. The AAI questionnaire is assessed for "coherence of statement" and "coherence of mind", with disjunctions of attachment (as in trauma) a usual cause of incoherence of statements about feelings. Thus experimental psychology, informed by attachment theory, operates in the same area of anxiety detection and control first seen in religious confession and autobiographies by persons hoping for relief from depressions and other aberrant emotional conditions. Does the AAI's carefully methodized "guided creativity" portend a loss of the spontaneity and inventiveness of literary and artistic creativity? Does it take away from the arcane wonders of traditional culture, democratizing and cheapening what formerly only a few had access to? Of course the AAI is a little-known instrument of assessment used mainly by researchers, but it is part of a healthy wide-spread urge to discover hidden feelings in the interest of lessening trauma—especially in raising children. From the "rap groups" of traumatized Vietnam veterans to the sometimes unseemly disclosures of talk shows, there is a powerful movement to understand the effects and sources of emotional suffering. Is culture being debased? I do not think so. If "mass confessional creativity" helps to remove the causes of infant and childhood anxious attachments, we will be so well served as to lessen the lament for fewer expressive arts distinguished by esoteric aestheticism. As awareness gathers of creativity originating with anxious attachments, art will be enriched, not cheapened nor disappear. The arts may become more therapeutically aware, quicker to identify damaging and reparative imageries, but that may well enhance their healing function.

There is no escaping psychologies of creativity; to talk about the arts without them is like discussing physics with no theory of matter and energy. The problem is to find, or to synthesize, the best theory of creativity—the one fitting most cases of how motivating energies in gifted persons bring about artistic products. The debate this century within psychoanalysis, and other psychologies, has been protracted and remains incomplete. We have surveyed the pioneering contentions of Freud, Rank, Klein, Fairbairn, Winnicott, Stokes, Milner and Miller in the hope of finding agreements. The common theme is anxiety as a prime motivation in creativity, but there is no consensus as to how anxiety arises developmentally, and how it is said to work depends on the degree to which Freudian drive theory is favored over an object relations theory of how persons develop and interact. The shift in psychoanalysis towards an object relations theory of personality formation, due largely to Fairbairn, has reoriented thinking about creativity to mother-infant developmental relatedness and internalizations by the infant of its negative features. But we have gone beyond both drive theory and object relations to ask for consideration of attachment theory as the starting point for the most accurate thinking about how anxiety enters psycho-physical systems and creativity arises to reduce its stressfulness.

John Bowlby had little to say about the arts, and creativity is strangely missing from his formulation of human development as guided by instinctive attachment behavior. I have tried to work out what Bowlby might have said about creativity had he put his mind to it. While Bowlby's basic Darwinian tenet holds to observation of what actually goes on in nature, the scope of enquiry now extends well beyond the attachment and loss paradigm he proposed to a trauma-caused paradigm of emotional disorder. Bowlby, and his immediate followers, said less about child abuse than would be necessary today; theory of creativity, which must explain the manic-depressive, or dissociative dimension, therefore, has need of an expanded theory of attachment behavior. Such a comprehensive theory is just coming into view, especially in the work of Patricia Crittenden, which is admittedly speculative beyond the strict empiricism observed by Bowlby.

Nonetheless, Bowlby's broad formulation of the origin of anxious attachments rings true. Conditions activating anxious attachment in infants are of three major types: environmental such as alarming events and rebuffs by adults or other children; conditions within the attachment relationship, such as absence, departure, or discouragement of proximity on the part of the caregiver; and conditions of the child, such as fatigue, hunger, pain and sickness.[26] Each, in some combination, bears on the child's need to take creative measures for survival. Sometimes, as can be psychobiographically reconstructed, these anxiety-causing conditions lead along a scale of adaptation to formal endeavors in the creative arts. Thus understanding of how fundamental to life attachments actually are orients us towards a unified theory of creativity. The arts may offer only a comforting illusion of transcending human ills, or they can be more closely examined for commentary on how we strive beyond anxiety for a sense of secure being. To take the latter view need not be reductionist, as long as the reparative transcendence of art is also remembered.

Occasionally an artist has recognized this and put it in words. The painter Paul Klee, one of the most imaginatively gifted in this century, is reported to have said, "At the highest level, imagination is guided by instinctual stimuli, and illusions are created which buoy us up and stir us more than do the familiar things of earth. In that realm are born the symbols which comfort the mind, which perceives that it need not be chained to the potentialities of terrestrial things".[27] Attachment and transcendence can sometimes cohere.

Notes

1. Robert Burton, *The Anatomy of Melancholy*, ed. Holbrook Jackson (London: J. M. Dent, 1932), vol. 2, p. 120. Rainer Maria Rilke, *Duino Elegies*, tr. O. F. MacIntyre (Berkeley: University of California Press, 1961), p. 3.

2. See Sidra Stich, *Anxious Visions: Surrealist Art*. (New York: Abbeville Press, 1990), p. 74f.

3. Myron A. Hofer, "Early Symbiotic Processes: Hard Evidence From a Soft Place," in *Pleasure Beyond the Pleasure Principle*, ed. Robert A. Glick and Stanley Bone (New Haven: Yale University Press, 1990), p. 59.

4. Ibid., p. 62.

5. Myron A. Hofer, "Hidden Regulators: Implications for a New Understanding of Attachment, Separation and Loss," in *Attachment Theory: Social, Developmental and Clinical Perspectives*, ed. Susan Goldberg, Roy Muir and John Kerr (Hillsdale, N.J.: The Analytic Press, 1995), p. 224. To "hidden regulators" should be added C. Waddington's idea of "self righting", an embryological concept, which describes "an inherent tendency to recover or rebound from a developmental deficit with a developmental progression as a result of positive change in an inhibiting external condition" (in Allan N. Schore, *Affect Regulation and the Origin of the Self: The Neurobiology of Emotional Development* (Hillsdale, N.J.: Lawrence Erlbaum, 1994), p. 464).

6. Ibid., p. 221.

7. Allan N. Schore, *Affect Regulation and the Origin of the Self*, p. 358. For discussion of these preverbal processes see pp. 389–90.

8. Ibid., p. 361. Schore cites Carroll E. Izzard's view "that repressed shame obviates self-repair", quoting Izzard that "the effort to repair and strengthen the self after experiencing intense shame" is a powerful but often frustrated motive, p. 362. Izzard's most notable work is on "Facial Expression and the Regulation of Emotions," *Journal of Personality and Social Psychology*, 58, no. 3 (1990): 487-498. For the importance of the mother's face and facial interactions with the infant in generating and controlling shame see Ana-Maria Rizzuto, "Shame in Psychoanalysis. The Function of Unconscious Fantasies," *International Journal of Psycho-Analysis*, 72 (1991): 297-312.

9. Marvin Eisenstadt et al., *Parental Loss and Achievement* (Madison, CT: International Universities Press, 1989); Andrew Brink, *Obsession*

and Culture: A Study of Sexual Obsession in Modern Fiction (Madison/ Teaneck, N.J.: Fairleigh Dickinson University Press, 1996).

10. Carol M. Ravenal, "Three Faces of Mother: Madonna, Martyr, Medusa in the Art of Edvard Munch," *Journal of Psychohistory*, 13, no. 4 (1986): 383.

11. Mary Mathews Gedo, *Picasso: Art as Autobiography* (Chicago: University of Chicago Press), p. 9. Picasso's school phobia and learning block are studied as narcissistic reactions to separation from his father, pp. 14-15.

12. Frances Spalding, "Expressions of Universal Evil," review of Andrew Sinclair, *Francis Bacon: His Life and Violent Times*, *The Times Literary Supplement*, September 24, 1993, p. 17.

13. Margaret Mitscherlich-Nielsen, "Psychoanalytic Notes on Franz Kafka: The Psychobiography of a Disturbed Genius," *Psychocultural Review*, 3, no.1 (1979):1–23. Ronald Hayman, *Kafka: A Biography* (New York: Oxford University Press, 1982).

14. Kenneth S. Lynn, *Hemingway* (New York: Simon and Schuster, 1987), p. 10.

15. See for instance Irvin D. and Marilyn Yalom, "Ernest Hemingway—a Psychiatric View," *Archives of General Psychiatry*, 24, June (1971): 485–94; Michael L. Fleisher, "Twin Fantasies, Bisexuality and Creativity in the Works of Ernest Hemingway," *International Review of Psycho-Analysis*, 16 (1990): 287–98.

16. Deirdre Bair, *Samuel Beckett: A Biography* (London: Jonathan Cape, 1978); Didier Anzieu, "Beckett and Bion," *International Review of Psycho-Analysis*, 16 (1989): 163–69; Bennett Simon, "The Imaginary Twins: The Case of Beckett and Bion," *International Review of Psycho-Analysis*, 15 (1988):332–52.

17. Linda Hutcheon, *Formalism and the Freudian Aesthetic: the Example of Charles Mauron* (Cambridge: Cambridge University Press, 1984), pp. 1-13. Mauron (d. 1966) was limited by reading only Freud, Melanie

Klein and Adrian Stokes (see pp. 128, 192); nonetheless Mauron's method of contacting the author's unconscious by systematically collecting "obsessive metaphors" had much to recommend it. Leonard Shengold emphasizes the importance of understanding metaphor as a means of helping victims of child abuse. (See *Soul Murder: The Effects of Childhood Abuse and Deprivation* (New York: Ballantine Books, 1991), p. 297. Verbal and visual imagery analysis of political cartoons and statements has been highly developed by Lloyd de Mause and other psychohistorians.

18. William Wordsworth, *The Prelude*, ed. J. O. Maxwell (Harmondsworth: Penguin Books,1972), pp. 52, 55. The novelist Virginia Woolf was equally definite about her hope for emotional healing. After saying that it is a "shock receiving capacity" that makes her a writer, Woolf speaks of the novel as "a token of some real thing behind appearances; and I make it real by putting it into words. It is only by putting it into words that I make it whole; this wholeness means that it has lost its power to hurt me; it gives me, perhaps because by doing so I take away the pain, a great delight to put the severed parts together ("A Sketch of the Past," in Virginia Woolf, *Moments of Being*, ed. Jeanne Schulkind. New York: Harcourt Brace Jovanovich, 1976, p.72.) Woolf wrote these words in 1939; as is well known, she was overtaken by suicidal despair, ending her life in 1941. There is debate over the extent to which early sexual abuse contributed to Woolf's adult emotional disorder.

19. For background see Jeffrey Berman, *The Talking Cure: Literary Representations of Psychoanalysis* (New York: New York University Press, 1987), chapter 1. Novel writing as therapeutic narrative is studied by Barbara and Richard Almond in *The Therapeutic Narrative: Fictional Relationships and the Process of Psychological Change* (Westport, CT: Praeger, 1996).

20. James W. Pennebaker et al., "Disclosure of Traumas and Immune Function: Health Implications for Psychotherapy," *Journal of Consulting and Clinical Psychology*, 56, no. 2 (1988): 239–45. See also B. Perry "Neurobiological Sequelae of Childhood Trauma: PTSD

in Children," in M. Marburg, ed., *Catecholamine Function in Post Traumatic Stress Disorder: Emerging Concepts*. (Washington, D.C.: American Psychiatric Press, 1994), pp. 233–55.

21. Judith L. Herman, *Trauma and Recovery* (New York: Basic Books, 1992), p. 42.

22. James W. Pennebaker, *Opening Up : The Healing Power of Expressing Emotions* (New York: The Guilford Press, 1997), p. 178. Use of expressive art and writing in reducing the anxiety of traumas is increasingly recognized among analysts. See, for example, Pirkko L. Graves "Life Event and Art," *International Review of Psycho-Analysis,* 11, (1984): 76 and Dori Laub and Daniel Podell, "Art and Trauma," *International Journal of Psycho-Analysis*, 355–65; (1995): 991–1005. Ernst Kris was among the earliest analytic writers on the arts to call attention to "traumatic experience which, long repressed, still exercises influences" upon the wish to create artistic objects *Psychoanalytic Explorations in Art* (London: George Allen & Unwin, 1953), p. 33.

23. Ibid., p. 186.

24. B. A. van der Kolk and Onno van der Hart, "The Intrusive Past: the Flexibility of Memory and the Engraving of Trauma," *American Imago*, 48, no. 4 (1991): 450.

25. Joshua Kendall, "Advances in Diagnosing and Treating Dissociative Disorders," *Treating Abuse Today*, March-April, (1997): 17f. See also *Treating Dissociative Identity Disorder* ed. James L. Spira (San Francisco: Jossey-Bass Publishers, 1996) for the importance of expressive therapies using play, art and writing to allow abused children to maintain verbal silence while expressing feelings. See especially p. 244f.

26. John Bowlby, *Attachment and Loss* (London: The Hogarth Press, 1969), vol. 1, *Attachment*, pp. 258-59.

27. Felix Klee, *Paul Klee*, tr. R. and C. Winston (New York: George Braziller, 1962), p. 155. Paul Klee caught the European inter-war mood

of fear and apprehension in such pictures as *Mask of Fear* (1932), *Fear* (1934). and *Death and Fire* (1940), but Klee's reparative art far transcends these foreboding pictures.

Bibliography

Selected Books and Monographs

Almond, Barbara and Richard Almond. *The Therapeutic Narrative: Fictional Relationships and the Process of Psychological Change.* Westport, CT: Praeger, 1996.

Anthony, E. J. and T. Benedek, eds. *Depression and Human Existence.* Boston: Little Brown, 1975.

Arieti, Silvano MD and Jules Bemporad MD. *Severe and Mild Depression: The Psychotherapeutic Approach.* New York: Basic Books, 1978.

Art Gallery Council of Great Britain. *Catalogue to Adrian Stokes Retrospective.* Serpentine Gallery London:1982.

Augustine, Saint. *Confessions.* Translated by E. B. Pusey. London: Dent, 1957.

Babb, Lawrence. *The Elizabethan Malady: A Study of Melancholia in English Literature from 1580–1642.* East Lansing: Michigan State University Press, 1951.

Bair, Dierdre. *Samuel Beckett: A Biography.* London: Jonathan Cape, 1978.

Beckett, Samuel. *Company.* London: Picador/Pan Books. 1982.

——. *Eleutheria,* London: Faber, 1996.

——. *A Dream of Fair to Middling Women.* Dublin: Black Cat, 1992.

——. *Waiting for Godot.* New York: Grove Press, 1954.

——. *Endgame.* New York: Grove Press, 1958.

Belmaker, R.H. and H.M. van Praag, eds. *Mania: An Evolving Concept.* SP Medical & Scientific Books, 1980.

Benson, Herbert. *The Relaxation Response.* London: Collins, 1976.

Berman, Jeffrey. *The Talking Cure: Literary Representations Of Psychoanalysis.* New York: New York University Press, 1987.

Bonaparte, Marie. *The Life and Work of Edgar Allen Poe: A Psycho-Analytic Interpretation.* London: Imago Publishing, 1933.

Bowlby, John. *A Secure Base: Clinical Applications of Attachment Theory.* London: Routledge, 1988.

——. *Attachment and Loss.* 3 Vols. London: Hogarth Press, 1969, 1973, 1980.

Brain, Russell. *Some Reflections on Genius and Other Essays.* London: Pitman, 1960.

Brazleton, T. Berry and Michael W. Yogman. *Affective Development in Infancy.* Norwood, NJ: Ablex, 1986.

Brink, Andrew. *Obsession and Culture: A Study of Sexual Obsession in Modern Fiction.* Madison/ Teaneck, NJ Fairleigh Dickinson University Press, 1996.

Brown, George W. and Tirril Harris. *Social Origins of Depression: A Study of Psychiatric Disorder.* New York: The Free Press, 1978.

Bunyan, John. *Grace Abounding to the Chief of Sinners.* Edited by Roger Sharrock.. Oxford: Clarendon Press, 1962.

Burton, Robert. *The Anatomy of Melancholy.* Edited by H. Jackson. London: J. M. Dent, 1961.

Cannon, Walter B. *The Wisdom of the Body.* New York: W.W. Norton, 1939.

Cardinal, Marie. *The Words to Say It.* Cambridge, MA: VanVactor & Goodheart, 1983.

Claridge, Gordon. et al., *Sounds from the Bell Jar: Ten Psychotic Authors* (London: Macmillan, 1990).

Clegg, Hugh Griffith. *The Reparative Motif in Child and Adult Therapy.* New York: Jason Aronson, 1984.

Cohen, I. K. et al., eds. *Wound Healing: Biochemical & Clinical Aspects.* Philadelphia: W. B. Saunders, 1992.

Cousins, Norman. *Anatomy of an Illness: Reflections on Healing.* New York: W. W. Norton, 1979.

Cowper, William. *Poetical Works.* Edited by H.S. Milford, London: Oxford University Press, 1967.

Coyne, James C., ed. *Essential Papers on Depression.* New York University Press, 1986.

Cytryn, Leo, M.D. and Donald H. McKnew M.D. *Growing Up Sad: Childhood Depression and its Treatment.* New York: W. W. Norton, 1996.

Dante. *The Divine Comedy.* Translated by Dorothy L. Sayers. Harmondsworth: Penguin Books, 1949, 1955, 1962.

Darwin, Charles. *The Expression of Emotion in Man and Animals.* London: Murray, 1872.

De Salvo, Louise. *Virginia Woolf: The Impact of Childhood Sexual Abuse on Her Life and Work.* Boston: Beacon Press, 1989.

Dictionary of National Biography, vol. 1.

Dijkstra, Bram. *Idols of Perversity: Fantasies of Feminine Evil in Fin-du-Siècle Culture.* New York: Oxford University Press, 1986.

Dinsmore, Charles E. ed. *A History of Regeneration Research.* Cambridge University Press, 1991.

Donne, John. *The Complete English Poems.* Edited by A. J. Smith. London: Penguin, 1971.

Dreifuss-Kattan, Esther. *Cancer Stories: Creativity and Self-Repair.* Hillsdale, NJ: The Analytic Press,1990.

Dunn, Douglas. *Elegies.* London: Faber and Faber, 1985.

Eisenstadt, Marvin et al. *Parental Loss and Achievement.* Madison, CT: International Universities Press, 1989.

Ellenberger, Henri F. , *The Discovery of the Unconscious: The History and Evolution of Dynamic Psychiatry.* London: Allen Lane, 1970.

Ellis, Havelock. *A Study of British Genius.* London: Hurst and Blackett, 1904.

Emde, Robert N. et al., *Emotional Expression in Infancy: A Biobehavorial Study, Psychological Issues*, 10, no.1, Monograph 37. New York: International Universities Press, 1974.

Fairbairn, W.R.D. *From Instinct to Self: Selected Papers of W.R.D. Fairbairn.* Edited by E. F. Birtles and D. E. Scharff. Northvale, NJ: Jason Aronson, 1994.

——. *Psychoanalytic Studies of the Personality.* London: Tavistock, 1952.

Ferenczi, Sandor. *The Clinical Diary of Sandor Ferenczi.* Edited by J. Dupont. Harvard University Press, 1988.

Fielding, Henry. *Tom Jones.* Edited by Sheridan Baker. New York: Norton, 1995.

Fincino, Marsilio. *De Vita Libri Tres. Opera Omnia.* 2 Vols. Turin: Bottega d'Erasmo, 1962.

Fox, George. *The Journal of George Fox.* Edited by John Nickalls. Cambridge University Press, 1952.

Fraser, Sylvia. *My Father's House.: A Memoir of Incest and Healing.* Toronto: Doubleday Canada, 1987.

Freud, Sigmund. *Collected Papers.* Edited by Joan Riviere. New York: Basic Books, 1957.

——. *Standard Edition of the Complete Psychological Works of Sigmund Freud.* Edited by James Strachey. London: Hogarth Press, 1963.

Freyd, Jennifer J. *Betrayal Trauma: The Logic of Forgetting Childhood Abuse*. Harvard University Press, 1996.

Fuller, Peter. *Art and Psychoanalysis.* London: Writers and Readers Cooperative, 1980.

Garber, Marjorie. *Vice Versa: Bisexuality and Eroticism in Everyday Life.* New York: Simon and Schuster, 1995.

Gedo, Mary Mathews. *Picasso: Art as Autobiography.* Chicago: University of Chicago Press, 1980.

Glick, Robert A., and Stanley Bone, eds. *Pleasure Beyond the Pleasure Principle*. New Haven:Yale University Press, 1990.

Goldberg, Susan, Roy Muir and John Kerr., eds. *Attachment Theory, Social, Developmental, and Clinical Perspectives.* Hillsdale, NJ: The Analytic Press, 1995.

Goodwin, Fredrick K. and Kay R. Jamison. *Manic-Depressive Illness.* New York: Oxford University Press, 1990.

Grohman,Will. *Paul Klee*. New York: Abrams, n.d.

Grosskurth, Phyllis. *Byron: The Flawed Angel*. Toronto: Macfarlane Walter & Ross, 1997.

Grotstein, J. S. and D. B. Rinsley, eds. *Fairbairn and the Origins of Object Relations.* New York: Guilford, 1994.

Guntrip, Harry. *Schizoid Phenomena, Object-Relations and the Self.* London, Hogarth, 1968.

Gut, Emmy. *Productive and Unproductive Depression: Success or Failure of a Vital Process.* New York: Basic Books, 1989.

Hamilton, Ian. *Robert Lowell: A Biography.* New York: Vintage, 1983.

Hardy, Thomas. *The Complete Poetical Works*. Edited by Samuel Hynes. Oxford: Clarendon Press, 1995.

Hayman, Ronald. *Kafka: A Biography.* New York: Oxford University Press, 1982.

Hemingway, Ernest. *The Garden of Eden.* New York: Charles Scribner's Sons, 1986.

Herbert, George. *The Works.* Edited by F.E. Hutchinson. Oxford: Clarendon Press, 1959.

Herman, Judith L. *Trauma and Recovery.* New York: Basic Books, 1992.

Hesse, Hermann. *Autobiographical Writings.* New York: Farrar, Straus and Giroux, 1972.

Holbrook, David. *Sylvia Plath: Poetry and Existence.* London: Athlone, 1976.

Holmes, Jeremy. *John Bowlby and Attachment Theory.* London: Routledge, 1993.

Hutcheon, Linda. *Formalism and the Freudian Aesthetic: the Example of Charles Mauron.* Cambridge: Cambridge University Press, 1984.

Jamison, Kay Redfield. *Touched with Fire: Manic Depressive Illness and the Artistic Temperment.* New York: The Free Press, 1993.

——. *An Unquiet Mind.* New York: Alfred A. Knopf, 1995.

Jones, Ernest. *The Life and Work of Sigmund Freud.* Edited by L. Trilling and S. Marcus, London: Pelican, 1964.

Jung, C. G. *Memories, Dreams and Reflections.* Edited by Aniela Jaffé. New York: Vintage Books, 1965.

Kafka, Franz. *The Castle.* Translated by Willa and Edwin Muir. New York: Knopf, 1968 [c1954].

——. *The Trial.* Translated by Willa and Edwin Muir. New York: Schocken Books, 1968 [c1956].

——. *The Basic Kafka.* Edited by Erich Heller. New York: Pocket Books, 1979.

Kahr, Brett. *D. W. Winnicott, A Biographical Portrait.* Madison, CT: International Universities Press, 1996.

Kandinsky, Wassily . *Concerning the Spiritual in Art and Painting in Particular.* New York: George Wittenborn, 1955.

Kavaler-Adler, Susan. *The Compulsion to Create: A Psychoanalytic Study of Women Artists* . New York: Routledge, 1993.

——. *The Creative Mystique: From Red Shoes Frenzy to Love and Creativity.* New York: Routledge, 1996.

King, Henry. *The Poems.* Edited by Margaret Crum. Oxford: Clarendon Press, 1965.

Klee, Paul. *The Diaries, 1898–1918.* Edited by Felix Klee. University of California Press, 1964.

——. *On Modern Art.* London: Faber, 1948.

Klee, Felix. *Paul Klee.* Translated by R. and C. Winston. New York: George Braziller, 1962.

Klein, Melanie. *Envy and Gratitude and Other Works,* 1946–1963. New York: Delta, 1977.

——. *Love, Guilt and Reparation and Other Works, 1921–1945.* New York: Delta, 1977.

Kris, Ernst. *Psychoanalytic Explorations in Art.* London: George Allen & Unwin, 1953.

Laski, Marghanita. *Ecstasy, a Study of Some Secular and Religious Experiences.* London: Crescent Press, 1971.

Lear, Frances. *The Second Seduction.* New York: Alfred A. Knopf, 1992.

Leder, M.H., ed. *Anxiety.* London: Headley, 1969.

Lombroso, Cesare. *The Man of Genius.* London: Walter Scott, 1891.

Lowell, Robert. *Life Studies.* New York: Farrar, Straus and Giroux, 1959.

Lynn, Kenneth S. *Hemingway.* New York: Simon and Schuster, 1987.

Malcolm, Janet. *In the Freud Archives.* New York: Vintage, 1985.

Marburg, M. ed. *Catecholamine Function in Posttraumatic Stress Disorder: Emerging Concepts.* Washington, D.C.: American Psychiatric Press, 1994.

Masson, Jeffery M. *Final Analysis: The Making and Unmaking of a Psychoanalyst.* Reading, Mass.: Addison-Wesley, 1990.

May, Rollo. *The Meaning of Anxiety.* New York: Ronald Press, 1950.

Meltzer, Donald and Meg Harris Williams. *The Apprehension of Beauty.* Perthshire: The Clunie Press for The Ronald Harris Library, no. 14, 1988.

Menaker, Lewis, ed. *Biologic Basis of Wound Healing.* New York: Harper & Row, 1975.

Middlebrook, Diane. *Anne Sexton: A Biography.* Boston: Houghton Mifflin, 1991.

Miller, Alice. *Banished Knowledge: Facing Childhood Injuries.* New York: Doubleday, 1990.

——. *The Drama of the Gifted Child* (1979). New York: Basic Books, 1990.
——. *For Your Own Good: Hidden Cruelty in Child-Rearing and the Roots of Violence.* New York: Farrar, Straus, and Giroux, 1983.
——. *Paths of Life: Seven Scenarios.* New York: Pantheon Books, 1998.
——. *Pictures of a Childhood: Sixty-six Watercolors and an Essay* New York: Farrar, Straus and Giroux, 1986.
——. *Thou Shalt Not Be Aware: Society's Betrayal of the Child.* New York: Meridian, 1986.
——. *The Untouched Key: Tracing Childhood Trauma in Creativity and Destructiveness* New York: Doubleday, 1990.
Milne, Lorus J. and Margery Milne, *The Ages of Life.* New York: Harcourt, Brace & World, 1968.
Milner, Marion. *Eternity's Sunrise: A Way of Keeping a Diary.* London: Virago, 1987.
——. (Joanna Field, pseud.) *An Experiment in Leisure.* (1937) Los Angeles: Jeremy Tarcher,1987.
——. (Joanna Field, pseud.) *A Life of One's Own.* (1934) London:Virago Press, 1986.
——. *The Hands of the Living God: An Account of a Psycho-Analytic Treatment.* New York: International Universities Press, 1969.
——. *On Not Being Able to Paint* (1950). London: Heinemann, 1971.
——. *The Suppressed Madness of Sane Men: Forty-four Years of Exploring Psychoanalysis.* London: Tavistock, 1987.
Milton, John. *The Poetical Works.* London: Oxford University Press, 1958.
Morgan, Thomas Hunt. *Embryology and Genetics.* New York: Columbia University Press, 1934.
——. *Regeneration.* New York: Macmillan, 1901.
Mrosovsky, Nicholas. *Rheostasis: The Physiology of Change.* New York: Oxford University Press, 1990.
Naevestad, Marie. *The Colors of Rage and Love: The Process of Change in Psychotherapy Elucidated by the Patient's Own Drawings.* Oslo, Norway:Universitetsforlaget, 1979.
Oremland, Jerome D. *The Origins and Psychodynamics of Creativity: A Psychoanalytic Perspective.* Madison, CT: International Universities Press, 1997.

Pennebaker, James W. *Opening Up: The Healing Power of Expressing Emotions.* New York:The Guilford Press, 1997.

Phillips, Adam. *Winnicott.* London: Fontana, 1988.

Plath, Sylvia. *Ariel.* London: Faber, 1965.

——. *The Bell Jar.* London: Faber, 1966.

——. *The Journals.* Edited by Ted Hughes. New York: Dial Press, 1982.

——. *Letters Home: Correspondence 1950–1963.* New York: Harper and Row, 1975.

Polezhaev, L.V. *Loss and Restoration of Regenerative Capacity in Tissues and Organs of Animals.* Harvard University Press, 1972.

Pope, Alexander. *The Rape of the Lock.* In *The Poems.* Edited by John Butt. London: Methuen, 1963.

Porter, R. and J. Knight, eds. *Physiology, Emotion and Psychosomatic Illness.* Amsterdam: Elsevier-Excerpta, 1972.

Powles, William E. *Human Development and Homeostasis: the Science of Psychiatry.* Madison, CT: International Universities Press, 1992.

Rank, Otto. *Art and Artist: Creative Urge and Personality Development* (1932). New York: W. W. Norton, 1989.

——. *The Trauma of Birth* (1923). New York: Robert Brunner, 1952.

Rapee, R. M., ed. *Current Controversies in the Anxiety Disorders.* New York: The Guilford Press, 1996.

Rembrandt. *All the Etchings.* Edited by Gary Schwartz. London: Oresko Books, 1977.

Richards, Ruth L."Relationships Between Creativity and Psychopathology: An Evaluation and Interpretation of the Evidence." *Genetic Psychology Monographs* (Harvard Medical School) no. 103 (1981): 294.

Rieger, B. M., ed. *Dionysus in Literature: Essays on Literary Madness.* Bowling Green, OH: Bowling Green State University, Popular Press, 1994.

Rilke, Rainer Maria. *Duino Elegies.* Translated by O. F. MacIntyre. Berkeley: University of California Press, 1961.

——. *Letter to a Young Poet.* New York: W. W. Norton, 1963.

Roose, S.P. and R.A. Glick.,eds. *Anxiety as Symptom and Signal.* Hillsdale, NJ: The Analytic Press, 1995.

Rose, Gilbert J. *Trauma and Mastery in Life and Art.* New Haven, NJ: Yale University Press, 1987.

——. *The Power of Form: A Psychoanalytic Approach to Aesthetic Form.* Madison, CT: International Universities Press, 1992.

——. *Necessary Illusion: Art as Witness.* Madison, CT: International Universities Press, 1969.

Ross, Colin A. M.D. *The Osiris Complex: Case-Studies in Multiple Personality Disorder* Toronto :University of Toronto Press, 1994.

Rothenberg, Albert. *Creativity and Madness: New Findings and Old Stereotypes.* Baltimore: The Johns Hopkins University Press, 1990.

Rudnytsky, Peter L. *Transitional Objects and Potential Spaces: Literary Uses of D. W. Winnicott.* New York: Columbia University Press, 1993.

Schore, Allan N. *Affect Regulation and the Origin of the Self: The Neurobiology of Emotional Development.* Hillsdale, N J: Lawrence Erlbaum, 1994.

Segal, Hanna. *Dream, Phantasy and Art.* London and New York: Tavistock/ Routledge, 1991.

Sexton, Anne. *Anne Sexton: A Self-Portrait in Letters.* Edited by Linda Sexton and Lois Ames, Boston: Houghton Mifflin, 1977.

——. *The Death Notebooks.* Boston: Houghton Mifflin, 1974.

Sheldrake, Rupert. *A New Science of Life: The Hypothesis of Formalist Causation.* London: Granada, 1983.

Shengold, Leonard. *Soul Murder: The Effects of Childhood Abuse and Deprivation.* New York: Ballantine Books, 1991.

Spira, James L., ed. *Treating Dissociative Identity Disorder.* San Francisco: Jossey-Bass Publishers, 1996.

Stern, Daniel N. *The Interpersonal World of the Infant: A View from Psychoanalysis and Developmental Psychology.* New York: Basic Books, 1985.

Stettbacher, J. Konrad. *Making Sense of Suffering: The Healing Confrontation with Your Own Past.* New York: Dutton,1991.

Stevenson, Anne. *Bitter Flame: A Life of Sylvia Plath.* New York: Viking, 1989.

Stich, Sidra. *Anxious Visions: Surrealist Art.* New York: Abbeville Press, 1990.

Stokes, Adrian. *The Image in Form: Selected Writings of Adrian Stokes.* Edited by R. Wollheim, Harmondsworth: Penguin, 1972.

——. "Form in Art" In *New Directions in Psycho-Analysis*. Edited by Melanie Klein et al. New York: Basis Books, 1955.

——. *Reflections on the Nude*. London: Tavistock, 1967.

——. *Smooth and Rough*. London: Faber and Faber, 1951.

——. *Three Essays on the Painting of Our Time*. London: Tavistock, 1961.

——. *The Image in Form: Selected Writings*. Edited by Richard Wollheim. Harmondsworth: Penguin Books, 1972.

Styron, William. *Darkness Visible: A Memoir of Madness*. New York: Random House, 1990.

Sutherland, John D. *Fairbairn's Journey Into the Interior*. London: Free Association Books, 1989.

Thompson, D'Arcy. *On Growth and Form*. Cambridge University Press, 1961.

Trautmann, U., ed. *The Healing Arts in Dialogue*. Carbondale: Southern Illinois Press, 1981.

van der Kolk, Bessel A. et al. *Traumatic Stress: The Effects of Overwhelming Experience on Mind, Body, and Society*. New York: Guilford Press, 1996

Vaughan, Henry. *The Works*. Edited by L. C. Martin. Oxford: Clarendon Press, 1957.

Vernon, P.E., ed. *Creativity: Selected Readings*. Harmondsworth: Penguin, 1970.

Volkan, Vamik D. *Linking Objects and Linking Phenomena*. New York: International Universities Press, 1981.

Waddington, C.H. *Organizers and Genes*. Cambridge University Press, 1947.

Whyte, Lancelot Law. *Accent on Form: An Anticipation of the Science of Tomorrow*. Westport, CT: Greenwood Press, 1973.

Winnicott, Clare et al., eds. *Psycho-Analytic Explorations*. London: Karnac Books, 1989.

Winnicott, D.W. *The Maturational Processes and the Facilitating Environment*. London: Hogarth Press, 1965.

——. *The Piggle: An Account of the Psychoanalytic Treatment of a Little Girl*. New York: International Universities Press, 1977.

——. *Playing and Reality*. London: Tavistock, 1971.

——. *The Spontaneous Gesture: Selected Letters of D. W. Winnicott*. Edited by F. R. Rodman. Harvard University Press, 1987.

——. *Through Paediatrics to Psycho-Analysis*. London: Hogarth Press,1975.

Wirt, R. et al., eds. *Life History Research in Psychopathology*. Minneapolis: University of Minnesota Press, 1974.

Woolf, Virginia. *Moments of Being*. Edited by Jeanne Schulkind. New York: Harcourt Brace Jovanovich, 1976.

Wordsworth, William. *The Prelude*. Edited by J.O. Maxwell. Harmondsworth: Penguin Books, 1972.

Wright, Kenneth. *Vision and Separation between Mother and Baby*. Northvale, NJ :Jason Aronson, 1991.

Articles

Akiskal, H. S. and K. Akiskal. "Reassessing the Prevalence of Bipolar Disorders: Clinical Significance and Artistic Creativity." *Psychiatrie et Psychobiographie* 3 (1988).

Almasi, Lenato J. "The Face-Breast Equation." *Journal of the American Psychoanalytic Association* 8 (1960): 43.

Andreasen, Nancy and Arthur Canter. "The Creative Writer: Psychiatric Symptoms and Family History." *Comprehensive Psychiatry* 15, no. 2 (1974): 126.

Andreasen, Nancy. "Creativity and Mental Illness: Prevalence Rates in Writers and Their First-Degree Relatives." *American Journal of Psychiatry* 144: (1987):1290.

Andreasen, Nancy and Pauline Powers. "Creativity and Psychosis: An Examination of Conceptual Style." *Archives of General Psychiatry* 32 (1975):70.

Anon. "Interview with Alice Miller." *Omni*, March 1987, 80.

Anon. *Psychology Today* March/April, 1996, 11.

Anzieu, Didier. "Beckett and Bion." *International Review of Psycho-Analysis* 16 (1989): 163.

C.H. "Manic Depression and Creativity." *Science* 233 (1986): 725.

Chasseguet-Smirgel, Janine. "Thoughts on the Concept of Reparation and the Hierarchy of Creative Acts." *International Revew of Psycho-Analysis* 11 (1984): 399.

Cohen, Mabel Blake, et al. "An Intensive Study of Twelve Cases of Manic-Depressive Psychosis." *Psychiatry* 17 (1954): 120.

De Vries, Marco J. "Healing and the Process of Healing.", *Humane Medicine* 1, no.2 (1985): 57.

Dinnage, Rosemary. "Review of The Piggle." *Times Literary Supplement* Sept. 15, 1978, 1025.

Drevdahl, John E. and Raymond B. Cattell, "Personality and Creativity in Artists and Writers.", *Journal of Clinical Psychology* 14 (1958): 107.

Fairbairn, W.R.D. "Prolegomena to a Psychology of Art." *The British Journal of Psychology* 28 part 3 (1938).

——. "Synopsis of an Object-Relations Theory of the Personality." *International Journal of Psycho-Analysis* 44 no. 2 (1963):224–25.

——. "The Ultimate Basis of Aesthetic Experience" *British Journal of Psychology* 28, part 3 (1938).

Ferenczi, Sandor. "Confusion of Tongues Between Adults and the Child." *International Journal of Psycho-analysis* 30(1949): 225.

Fleisher, Michael L. "Twin Fantasies, Bisexuality and Creativity in the Works of Ernest Hemingway." *International Review of Psycho-Analysis,* 16, (1990): 287.

Fordham, Michael "A Reaction." *British Journal of Medical Psychology* 24 (1951): 72.

Gerend, Linda. "Moments of Delight." *Times Literary Supplement,* December 19, 1986, 119.

Gibson, Robert W., Mabel B. Gibson, and Robert A. Cohen. "On the Dynamics of the Manic Depressive Personality." *American Journal of Psychiatry* 115 (1959): 1102.

Graves, Pirkko L. "Life Event and Art." *International Review of Psycho-Analysis* 11 (1984): 355.

Grinberg, Leon, et al. "Panel on Creativity." *International Journal of Psycho-Analysis* 53 (1972): 21.

Hamilton, Ian. "The Embarrassing Pursuit." *Times Literary Supplement* April 29, 1994, p.17.

Holden, Constance. "Creativity and the Troubled Mind." *Psychology Today* April 1987: 9.

Isakower, O. "A Contribution to Patho-psychology of Phenomena Associated With Falling Asleep." *International Journal of Psycho-Analysis* 9, no.138 (1938):331.

Izzard, Caroll E. "Facial Expressions and the Regulation of Emotions." *Journal of Personality and Social Psychology* 58, no. 3 (1990): 487.

Jamison, Kay Redfield. "Clouds with Silver Linings: Positive Experiences Associated with Primary Affective Disorders." *American Journal of Psychiatry* 137, no. 2 (1980): 200.

——. "Mood Disorders and Patterns of Creativity in British Writers and Artists." *Psychiatry* 52 (1989): 131.

Juda, Adéle. "The Relationship Between Highest Mental Capacity and Psychic Abnormalities." *The American Journal of Psychiatry* 106, no. 1–12, (1949–50): 296.

Kanzer, Mark. "Writers and the Early Loss of a Parent." *Journal of the Hillside Hospital* 2, no. 3 (1953): 148–51.

Kendall, Joshua. "Advances in Diagnosing and Treating Dissociative Disorders." *Treating Abuse Today* March-April, (1997): 17.

Kendall, Joshua and Alan Plotkin. "Anne Sexton's Failed Psychotherapies: The Tragic Fate of 'Her Kind'." *Treating Abuse Today* 5, no. 2 (1995): 22.

Laub, Dori and Daniel Podell. "Art and Trauma." *International Journal of Psycho-Analysis* 76 (1995): 991.

Lichtenstein, Parker E. "Genius as Productive Neurosis." *The Psychological Record* 21(1971):151.

Mitscherlich-Nielsen, Margaret. "Psychoanalytic Notes on Franz Kafka: The Psychobiography of a Disturbed Genius." *Psychocultural Review,* 3, no. 1 (1979):1.

Pennebaker, James W. et al. "Disclosure of Traumas and Immune Function: Health Implications for Psychotherapy.", *Journal of Consulting and Clinical Psychology,* 56, no. 2 (1988): 239.

Pollock, George. "On Mourning, Immortality, and Utopia." *Journal of the American Psychoanalytic Association* 23 (1975): 334.

Post, Felix. "Creativity and Psychopathology: A Study of 291 World-Famous Men."*British Journal of Psychiatry* 165 (1994): 22.

Ravenal, Carol M. "Three Faces of Mother: Madonna, Martyr, Medusa in the Art of Edvard Munch." *Journal of Psychohistory* 13, no. 4 (1986): 383.

Rickman, John. "On the Nature of Ugliness and the Creative Impulse." *International Journal of Psycho-Analysis* 21 part 1 (1940): 308.

Riviere, Joan. "Magical Regeneration by Dancing." *International Journal of Psycho-Analysis* 11 (1930): 340.

Rizzuto, Ana-Maria. "Shame in Psychoanalysis. The Function of Unconscious Fantasies" *International Journal of Psycho-Analysis* 72 (1991): 297.

Simon, Bennett. "The Imaginary Twins: The Case of Beckett and Bion." *International Review of Psycho-Analysis* 15 (1988): 332.

Spalding, Frances. "Expressions of Universal Evil: A review of Andrew Sinclair's Francis Bacon: His Life and Violent Times." *The Times Literary Supplement* September 24, 1993, 17.

Stokes, Adrian. "Concerning Art and Metapsychology." *International Journal of Psycho Analysis* 26 (1945): 177.

——. "A Game That Must Be Lost." *International Journal of Psycho-Analysis.* 41 (1960):74.

—— Stokes, Adrian. "On Being Taken Out of Oneself." *International Journal of Psycho-Analysis,* 47(1966): 524.

Tronick, Edward Z. and Jeffery F. Cohn. "Infant-Mother Face-to-Face Interaction: Age and Gender Differences in Coordination and the Occurrence of Miscoordination." *Child Development* 60 (1989): 85–92.

van der Kolk, Bessel A. and Onno van der Hart. "The Intrusive Past: the Flexibility of Memory and the Engraving of Trauma." *American Imago* 48, no. 4 (1991): 450.

Winnicott, D.W. "Critical Notes." *British Journal of Medical Psychology* 24 (1951):76.

Wollheim, Richard. "Adrian Stokes, Critic Painter, Poet." *Times Literary Supplement* February 17, 1978, p. 207.

Wright, Kenneth. "Deep Calling Unto Deep: Artistic Creativity and the Maternal Object." *British Journal of Psychotherapy* 14, no. 4 (1998): 462.

Yalom, Irvin D. and Marilyn Yalom, "Ernest Hemingway—a Psychiatric View." *Archives of General Psychiatry* 24, June (1971): 485.

Name Index

THE RESHAPING OF PSYCHOANALYSIS
From Sigmund Freud to Ernest Becker

This series offers works that are concerned with the reshaping and revitalization of psychoanalysis. Also critical to this series is the interweaving of such disciplines as psychology, psychiatry, religion, and philosophy so as to promote dialogue and offer avenues toward rapprochement.

This series will publish and proffer studies of Freud and Neo-Freudians such as Becker, which are most aware of the long-term contributions of psychoanalysis toward the healing of self and society. Studies should be scholarly and clinically discerning. This is a series that is keenly concerned with the bridging of disciplines, the networking of ideas and peoples, and the perpetuation of the psychoanalytic questions, and, at times, its answers. This series is also very open to its authors' creativity and most appreciative of those efforts that reshape, revamp, revitalize, and transform Freudian psychoanalysis.

The general series editor is Barry R. Arnold, an Emory Ph.D., who is Associate Professor of Religious Studies and Philosophy at the University of West Florida. His area of specialty is psychoanalysis and medical ethics.

For additional information about this series or for the submission of manuscripts, please contact:

Peter Lang Publishing
Acquisitions Department
275 7th Avenue, 28th floor
New York, New York 10001

To order other books in this series, please contact our Customer Service Department:

(800) 770-LANG (within the U.S.)
(212) 647-7706 (outside the U.S.)
(212) 647-7707 FAX

Or browse online by series at:

www.peterlang.com

FSC
www.fsc.org
MIX
Papier | Fördert
gute Waldnutzung
FSC® C083411

Kolibri 360 GmbH
Ferdinand-Jühlke-Straße 7
99095 Erfurt, Deutschland
produktsicherheit@kolibri360.de

Druck:
CPI Druckdienstleistungen GmbH
im Auftrag der
Kolibri 360 GmbH
Ferdinand-Jühlke-Str. 7
99095 Erfurt